MW00893324

BORN WITH A BOMB

BORN WITH A BOMB

Suddenly Blind from Leber's Hereditary Optic Neuropathy

VALERIE BYRNE RUDISILL

Edited by Margie Sabol and Leslie Byrne

authorHOUSE®

AuthorHouse™
1663 Liberty Drive
Bloomington, IN 47403
www.authorhouse.com
Phone: 1-800-839-8640

© 2012 by Valerie Byrne Rudisill. All rights reserved.

No part of this book may be reproduced, stored in a retrieval system, or transmitted by any means without the written permission of the author.

Published by AuthorHouse   12/10/2012

ISBN: 978-1-4772-9585-4 (sc)
ISBN: 978-1-4772-9584-7 (hc)
ISBN: 978-1-4772-9586-1 (e)

Library of Congress Control Number: 2012922879

Any people depicted in stock imagery provided by Thinkstock are models, and such images are being used for illustrative purposes only.
Certain stock imagery © Thinkstock.

Because of the dynamic nature of the Internet, any web addresses or links contained in this book may have changed since publication and may no longer be valid. The views expressed in this work are solely those of the author and do not necessarily reflect the views of the publisher, and the publisher hereby disclaims any responsibility for them.

Front and back designed by Valerie Byrne Rudisll.

Front cover layout: Top left corner clockwise; Chase Rudisill with the Blue Man Group, Lawrence Byrne by Carl M Szabo Jr, James Crawford, Phoeng Gip, Catherine Knight, left to right - Estelle, George, and Elizabeth Stephan, Grant and Valerie Rudisill, Locke Milholland, David Rosser, Jeremy Poincenot, Jared Hara by Chyna Photography, Michell Gip.

For my family and friends whom have traveled along my side through grief and turmoil. For David, Chase Jacqui, Grant, and Larry life has been far from easy, I love you all. Finally, for all members of the LHON community, our family and friends, and the doctor's that are striving to help us.

A special thank you goes to each of the contributors who have made this book possible.

A portion of the proceeds from this collection goes toward research and each contributor.

I always knew looking back, the tears would make me laugh; but, I never knew looking back the laughs would make me cry.

Now I live every day as if it's my last.

David Rossner

Table of Contents

Contributed by Valerie Byrne Rudisill, Jared Hara, Locke Milholland, Jeremy Poincenot, Chase Rudisill, Leslie Byrne, Catherine Knight and Sandra Kanon, David Rossner (England), James Crawford(Australia), Lawrence Byrne, Phoeng Gip, Michell Gip, Valerie Byrne Rudisill, and Dr Edward Chu.

Welcome to our world

Walk a mile in our shoes

We sincerely hope you are not here to join us

The Paradigm Shift

Each person contributing to this collection has experienced a paradigm shift in their life. Each of us was forced to re-evaluate everything that comprised our current and future concept of our "life." In a matter of moments or months all that we knew changed, both for ourselves and also for each one of our beloved family members. This shift was far from a joyous enlightenment. It held the promise of life-altering tragedy, waiting to claim the eyesight of all maternally linked relatives at will and plunge us into darkness.

What follows is an introductory story and the stories of 12 people who have lost their eyesight. You will find humor, despair, courage, and inspiration throughout. The ages of the contributors range from 16 to late 50's. Each story is unique. None are professional writers. While a common theme exists, each story and style is different. Each one is told from deep within their souls. Some are funny, some are sad, some are serious. Each person provides inspiration, triumphing over one of the worst things life can throw you, being blind.

You will meet: Jared, in total darkness, but currently headed to the top of the music charts; Locke, a lawyer who is sure to entertain; Jeremy, the 2010 world blind golf champion; Chase, blind at 6 years old, but now 17 and visually impaired—doing amazinfeats and inspiring thore around him; George, who never knew he was part of our world; Catherine, who defied death; Locke, a lawyer who is sure to entertain; James from Australia, the longest-term blind contributor and avid sailor; David, from England, who survived a parachute not opening; Lawrence, a brilliant writer and musician; Phoeng, a survivor of the Cambodian Killing Fields; Michell, Phoeng's daughter who traveled to China in desperation for a cure and Grant, just 10 years old, the sole beholder of a hopeful future.

The Appendix contains a medical chapter by Dr. Edward Chu, which is a crash course in Leber's Hereditary Optic Neuropathy

*** **Please note: Chapter 8 is contributed by an English author and Chapter 9 is contributed by an Australian author. Due to this, the English contains slight variations.**

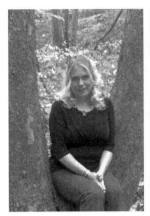
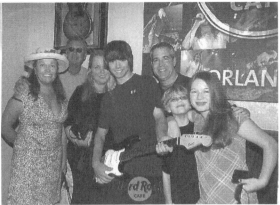

Sucker punch—Entering the World of LHON

In the summer of 1999, I received a phone call from my much younger 19 year old brother. He was not one to reach out so I was slightly surprised, but anticipated any sort of a normal conversation to ensue. My parents were traveling, so he was reaching out to me to determine the name of the ophthalmologist the family worked with. He wanted to know what day our parents would be home. I tried to send him to our optometrist (who provides glasses and lower level eye exams). He stopped me with a very, very shaky voice. He didn't need glasses. "Val, there is something extremely wrong with my eyes." I proceeded to contact our parents at their resort and set up an ophthalmology appointment coinciding with their return. I was a bit concerned, but my brother did have a flair for drama. For instance, a football injury would be believed to be a ruptured spleen that would lead to complete systemic failure, or a stubbed toe must also involve torn tendons and ligaments, etc.

With everything set on course, I went back to doing what I normally did, changing diapers or something. At the time I had a 3 ½ year old son and 1 ½ year old daughter. They needed me to do "stuff" for them. I needed to go do whatever mundane task was at hand, for I was blissfully unaware of the events that would follow. Meanwhile, we patiently waited for my brother's doctor appointment.

Upon my brother's return from the ophthalmologist's office, I received my next shaky voiced phone call. This time it was my mother, crying. This was no ruptured spleen. This was no stubbed toe. This did not involve glasses. The problem involved the optic nerves, the necessary parts of the body that carries the visual signal to the brain. Without the optic nerves, you are blind. That is it. Game over. No more sight. She said that they were not sure yet of the cause. It was possibly a brain tumor, some type of infection, Multiple Sclerosis, or maybe even genetic. Apparently the doctor had taken quite a pause when he took the extended families' medical history and learned my grandmother's brother had lost his sight during his mid twenties.

That evening, I tucked my children in bed. In their sweet little world, sugar plums were dancing in their heads, or maybe plastic dinosaurs were fighting, who knows. I was on a mission. I was more experienced than my parents at Internet research, so I hit the computer.

There are times in your life when you can get a complete sucker punch to the soul. When you know something really bad and in your gut you know it is the truth. The first punch, with two more to come, struck me within 30 minutes of computer researching: Leber's Hereditary Optic Neuropathy commonly referred to as LHON. It was bad, really, really bad. My brother was only at the beginning stage of losing his sight, more loss was sure to come. LHON was hereditary. It was a rare type of inheritance where all of a woman's offspring would carry something known as defective mitochondrial DNA. The father plays no role in the inheritance. Anyone maternally linked could lose their eyesight, at any time.

I looked in the mirror. This defective DNA may be coursing through my cells. I looked upstairs toward my children's rooms. It may be coursing through their cells, as well as my daughter's future children, my other brother, my mother, and the brother losing more vision with each passing day. There was absolutely no treatment. As I read and researched, my heart knew, we had this.

Patients, including my brother, undergo a variety of tests while doctors attempt to diagnose this problem. His MRI's were clear, and no brain tumors were present. There were no indications of Multiple Sclerosis. All tests were coming back normal as we waited for results of DNA testing. We were told this would take quite a while to get back because, well, criminal cases had all the labs working overtime. Lovely!

Eventually, the DNA test came back and we carried the genetic mutation #14484. My mother was distraught. She had been hoping for a brain tumor. They can be cut out, bombarded with radiation, something. For this nothing could be done. My brother was informed his vision should stop deteriorating at about 6-9 months, with a wide give or take on how severe it would be. He was also told he was young and had the best variety of the three primary mutations: 11778, 3460, and 14484. He was sure to regain some sight, carrying the 14484 mutation. He just needed to wait 18 months or so, again with a wide give or take on outcome, and he might be driving again. This part of the diagnosis he latched onto. He was determined to do the best he could to get through the next 18 months, and then pick up his life again.

As I would have conversations with my mother, she would cry. She relayed that things were bad for my brother. His sight was terrible. At this, my husband took a step backwards and said, "Well, sometimes things are exaggerated." I was not sold on his theory. Soon after, I saw my brother for the first time in a couple months. I was outside on the patio. We were having a dinner get together at my parents'. I watched my brother walk on the patio. He would gently place a foot in front of him, feel for any objects or unevenness, and then take a step. His short walk to the table was one of the longest, most painful walks I have ever witnessed. I was holding in tears. Next my mother brought him a plate and drink.

My brother had always been a proper and meticulous eater. Upon arrival of the plate, he lifted it while holding it an inch from his face. He was trying to locate the food on the plate. He then felt around for a fork and proceeded to eat with his face an inch or two from the plate. When searching for a drink, he fumbled slowly around until locating it. When he was finished, ¾ of the food was still on the plate. He thought he was done. So—that explained the 20 pounds he had lost since our last visit. My husband and I exchanged a glance. Holy shit!

At this point, my parents' and brother's journey to various neuro-ophthalmologists began. There was one about an hour away. There was one in Boston. There are probably a few other ones I don't recall. At this point in time, my information came either from the Internet or second hand through my families' visits. What we thought we knew was: Gene therapy was on the way, personally we had nothing to worry about. My kids were 4 and 2. The disease didn't strike until you were at least 17, giving an ample time-frame for the cure to arrive. I didn't need to worry about myself or my daughter because this hits males primarily. We chose to finish our family with a 3rd child, Grant, born in December of 2001. We were living in a misguided fantasyland.

Our first discovery that we may have some false information occurred when my brother hit the 18-month mark, at which time he was supposed to start getting some vision back. Weeks and months then passed. No improvement occurred. He slipped into a second round of depression that was of greater magnitude than the first. Before, he hung onto the hope of the ensuing recovery. As the known recovery window closed, so did his hope. This was permanent. There would be none of the promised driving. He would never get better. At this point I went back to my normal day to day routine, hoping for a new treatment for my brother and feeling content knowing that due to my children's ages, we would all be fine.

On an unbelievably gorgeous Saturday in May of 2002, we were roaming the fields of my oldest child, Chase's, school. Everyone was running, laughing, and giggling. They were a bunch of happy 6 year olds. Suddenly, the peace was broken by a shrilling scream following my deafening sobbing. The source of the clatter would be coming from my son, Chase. I grabbed his head and cradled him attempting to determine what had just happened. The source was a high speed impact injury to his right orbital bone, the outside of his eye socket. He was developing black eyes on both sides. His sister, 4, watched on scared over the drama. I looked at a friend, and said, "The scariest part of this is that we have this really rare eye disease and maybe this head trauma could cause him to go blind in his late teens."

Sucker punch number two. Within a week of the head injury, Chase began complaining his eyes weren't working right. Like his uncle, he had a flair for drama and he liked special attention. I told him he probably wasn't eating right and spaghetti had a lot of nutrition that would help his eyes. The next day, he said they were all better. The following day they were not working again. So I called my lifelong optometrist friend, Dr. Joanne Brilliant, and scheduled a next day appointment. I did not have much concern, as Leber's didn't happen to kids. I figured he knew his uncle had eye problems, and maybe wanted a little special attention with the new baby around.

We arrived at the appointment and proceeded to the machine that checks for nearsightedness. That test was fine. Next we went into the exam room and began the vision test. Chase told Dr. Jo, "My right eye isn't working so good." Dr. Jo started with his left eye and all was well. Then she went to the right eye. As she questioned what letter was on the wall, Chase responded with random guesses. She calmly kept enlarging the lines. After having no success with letters, Dr. Jo switched over to the largest available line for young kids, which involves airplanes, birthday cakes, etc. I am still holding onto to the attention seeking outcome. She asked what he sees and he responded again with random letters. Dr. Jo looks at Chase and says, "What if I told you it wasn't a letter?" Chase answered with a number. Immediately, heavy tears flowed from my eyes, fortunately concealed from my now one eye visioned son by the dark room. Had he been seeking attention he would have then guessed a false object. The logical thing to do if you can't actually see and you know it is not a letter, is to guess a number.

Suddenly my world imploded upon itself. I was flooded with fear, panic, disbelief, and adrenaline. My 6 year old was going blind, there is no cure, this doesn't happen to kids, and this can't be happening. Oh, but it was. I knew exactly the road we were about to travel down. Dear God No. He is only 6. This was a severe soul deep pain.

It was now our turn to walk my brother's path. You will often find a common theme among those with LHON, even with the prior genetic testing. We were sent to get MRI's, CAT scans, and blood tests. As predicted, all were normal. As we visited the neuro-ophthalmologist for the first time, my son took his first visual field tests. These are the most extremely boring tests known to mankind, searching for lights inside a white dome for an immeasurable amount of time while a person on the other end watches, via camera, as the subject slowly falls asleep. These tests are even difficult to endure even if you are an adult. Everyone I know hates them with a passion. So, I tried to make it fun. I called it the "shoot the alien test" and tried to convince my son it was like a video game. He did not buy into my theories. Yet, he did his very best and was a cooperative patient.

The tests showed severe center vision loss in his right eye and the left eye was beginning to show signs of deterioration. He would be blind in a couple months. There was a new open label trial going on with Alphagan-p, a glaucoma medication. The theory behind the study was that the medication was known to increase blood flow to the areas being affected, so maybe increased blood flow would help the cells survive.

So, at this point, we have our son's terrible field tests in our hands. We know he will soon be blind. The Dr. looks at us with a compassionate smile and says, "Oh don't worry, you have the best gene marker and he is young. He will recover his vision and be fine." If you notice, this is the same thing my brother was told. I just looked at him, thinking, "Whatever, should we go tell my brother this great news again? He will be so excited. Maybe that will make it true."

The follow up visits each contained worsening news. Chase's vision continued to deteriorate until he was counting fingers at 3 feet. The Alphagan-P did not show any success and the study was abandoned. It was time to do what many people do when diagnosed with a rare disease. Mainly, they fly to any specialist they find the name of. We flew to the Cleveland Eye center first. Then we went to see Dr. Nancy Nueman at the Emory Eye Center in Georgia. This was where our already demolished fantasyland became the badlands.

We learned many things on this visit. We discovered that Chase was not an anomaly and this disease did strike children, just not often. The bell curve runs something like age 1 to age 81. We learned there would be no gene therapy, at least not in the near future. If it came along, it would probably be in-uterus. (Please note that Bascom-Palmer is actively involved in current gene therapy research; our visit was 10 years ago.) We learned Chase would probably end up with 20/200 vision uncorrectable. We discovered the best hope potentially would come from nerve regeneration research that might be discovered in the effort to aide spinal cord injury victims. We learned that once he stabilized, his vision would remain unchanged (years later, we discovered this is another false pretense).

One particularly interesting thing we found out was that some researchers showed an interest in a supplement called Idebenone. This was not available in the United States at the time. So did we want to drive to Mexico, where you could get it, bring it across the border and give our 6 year old some Mexican produced, unregulated "supplement?" Heck no. In hindsight this may have been a good idea: Idebenone is currently showing some promise in studies. But we could not predict that and none of the doctors we saw recommended it. This was a harsh visit. Chase ended up blind in first and second grade. Yet luckily, he could still walk around and see his books using magnification.

What does one do for someone with a month or two of vision left? What does one do for a 6 year old losing their eyesight? Well, my first visit was to the library. I checked out about 20 pictorial books of magnificent places around the world. I thought maybe my son would somehow remember a few of the photos. Everything was quite crazy at that time and he already had trouble seeing books. No looking at the Great Wall of China for him. All this effort ultimately accomplished was a $173 late fine with the library. Several years later, they were kind enough to remove the fine when I explained the circumstances to library headquarters. They understood that returning the books was not on the forefront of my mind. Chase, of course, has no memory of the books.

What else can you do? Well, every kid wants to go to Disney World. My parents offered us a timeshare week they had. A co-worker at my husband's office actually had a fantastic contact at Disney. They made a few calls and they were able to procure four 5 day passes. Considering we were facing such stressful moments, every little thing helped. One thing we had discussed on the airplane to Florida was whether Chase had ever seen a rainbow. We discovered he had not and hoped one would show itself prior to extreme vision loss. By the grace of God, Chase saw a rainbow while walking down a long street at Universal Studios. Sometimes small things in life can make you feel really good inside.

One morning I was dropping Chase and his sister off at school when the school counselor ran over to my car and informed me I needed to come in at 10 a.m. for a meeting with no explanation available. Sorry, you can't say something like that and not explain what is going on. So I sat there, blocking the carpool line of 200 cars until I was able to discover the intent of the meeting. Hey, she is the one that chose the venue. Eventually, she gave in and informed me the school's intent was not to allow Chase to return the following year. It was a private school. We did not attend "their" 10 a.m. meeting, but scheduled a 9 a.m. the next day, including the school board and Church members I had notified of the meeting. The meeting was conducted by my husband, David, a highly skilled orator, who presented the attendees with 20 page informational packets on LHON.

At the time of the meeting, Chase was maintaining A's and B's. He had not incurred a singular behavioral referral and got along well with his peers. The school was concerned about us suing them. At that moment in time, the fear of a lawsuit was valid, but not before and not after their temporary decision. The first thing I did upon arriving home from carpool was to research the American's with Disabilities Act. Given the circumstances, should they refuse him attendance; I had the power to make their lives miserable. Anyhow, the meeting went according to David's plan and Chase spent many more comfortable years there.

Life settled back into "normal" mode and we each went about our daily lives. Chase is a fantastic athlete, sticking to running and a large white ball sport, also known as soccer. He cannot track lacrosse or baseballs and footballs blend in. He always did well at his academics, so complaining would be a crime.

Somehow, the stars aligned for my family, and Chase did regain much of his eyesight. He still has some missing spots in his vision and his optic nerves are 48% and 52% of normal thickness. However, what he does have left carries enough signals to his brain so that he qualifies for a driver's license. He is considered visually impaired. So that each of you feel comfortable, know that we were informed that not only did Chase qualify, but there are people with glaucoma and cataracts, etc., with much worse vision than him that also qualify. Think about that on your way out the door tomorrow. Shouldn't they have to have some orange flags on top of their car or something, so we can be extra careful around them? One comment I recently heard from Chase was, "Don't you have trouble figuring out where the stoplights are at an intersection?" Um, NO, I DON'T.

One thing I have not yet addressed is the feeling of isolation this disease originally presented. LHON is extremely rare with some estimates putting the affected U.S. population at around 4,000 people (out of 350,000,000 million). That does not include the carriers hanging out with their fingers crossed or blissfully unaware of its existence. When my brother and son went through their vision loss, there was no way of speaking to another person on the planet with the disease. Neither you, nor your "friends," will happen to know someone with it. There were no local or statewide organizations to join. Doctors could not give you another patient's phone number. You were totally alone, unless you had a relative you could ask questions and talk to.

Throughout his life, Chase was always much attuned to any changes in his vision. He would ask to get a visual field test (the shoot the alien test) whenever he felt his eyes were better or worse. He requested one in 6th grade and there was a decline in his vision. Recall, one thing we had learned at one visit to Emory was that this was not supposed to happen a second time. After several years off the computer, I was back on the research bandwagon. Ultimately, this action would be life-altering for me.

One thing I found while researching was a few medical articles on some patients who had gone through a second period of vision loss. So much for the safety of Chase's status as visually impaired versus blind. He could be "triggered" at any point and lose his current vision. Another thing I found was the existence of a many years long study, occurring in Brazil, on a several hundred person family that had the most common 11778 mutation, headed by Dr. Alfredo Sadun. I hoped one day to take Chase to Dr Sadun. The final, and ultimately life altering thing I discovered was a Yahoo group for people with LHON.

I immediately joined the Yahoo group and instantly we were no longer alone. There were other people. The isolation was over. Many of us checked in daily and we now had a core group of friends. We exchanged medical questions, we shared medical articles, and we discussed symptoms. More than this, we developed online friendships and would joke and kid with each other throughout the days. I am close to many of these people today and truly consider them my friends. After 7 years of being the only ones, this group was now a part of my life.

One of the members lived within driving distance of me in Maryland, another one was headed our way for business, and a third was planning to visit a friend nearby. Adding myself, the first group of LHON friends was planning a face to face meeting. This may sound mundane, but when something has affected your life to the extent Leber's Disease has affected ours, this is a really big deal. We were going to physically meet others with similar circumstances. Our excitement and joy was immeasurable. Two of the people from the dinner are actually now a very happy couple.

A while later a new member joined, Lissa Poincenot. Her son became affected and Lissa found herself a new purpose in life. She became one of the most LHON knowledgeable private individuals on the planet. Her job allows for travel and she has met people from all over the United States with LHON. Two Facebook groups had been formed, in addition to the Yahoo group, and Lissa personally reaches out to every person that joins.

On one of Lissa's trips to Maryland, she met up with me, my brother's wife, and a good, blind friend of ours. During this meeting, as we discussed various medical hopes for the future, Lissa made an off the cuff remark about a potential type of drop being developed which might help people actively losing their vision. This is vitally important later in the book.

At this point, everything once again had gone back to "normal." In my family, my grandmother had two brothers, one with LHON and one without. My mother had one brother, but he died in a car crash at the age of 24. I have two brothers, one with LHON and one without. The odds of a male with our mutation being affected hovers around 50%. While it does occur, women are much less likely to lose their vision. We had no affected females, so my family was doing a good job at following the statistical pie chart.

As you know, I have two boys and a girl. Given paper statistics, I had a base level of inner peace. Then, one evening my youngest son, Grant, at 8 years old tells me while playing in his room, "Mom, I can't see out of my right eye." Sucker punch number three. Grant's story is one you will not forget. He is pioneer for us all and provides hope for many aspects of the future. His is the final chapter of the book.

Valerie Byrne Rudisill

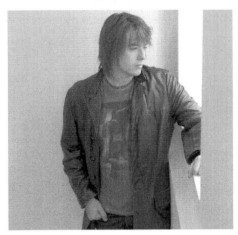
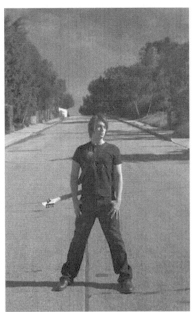

Blindsided

1 1 7 7 8. I wish this had been the combination to my hockey locker, or bike lock or even to my school locker. Instead, it was to be the combination to a genetic mutation at nucleotide position 11778 that would unlock a disease in my body at the age of eleven and would ultimately change my life forever.

My parents received the unimaginable call from the Mayo Clinic while I was attending the first day of school in 6th grade. That summer of 2003, I had gone to a hockey camp near the clinic in Rochester, Minnesota. Since I had lost vision in one eye and we were in the vicinity of what was one of the foremost clinics in the country, we thought maybe they could enlighten us as to what many other doctors before them could not: why I had lost vision in one eye. So after my two weeks in hockey camp, my father brought me to the Mayo Clinic for four days of tests before heading home to begin school. Even though the Mayo Clinic was unable to immediately give us a diagnosis, they were able to rule out anything life threatening, which was very comforting.

"Mr. Hara, is your wife there? This is Dr. Rho from Mayo. We just received your son's blood work back and I wanted to tell you both what was found." My father got my mother on the other line and with great anticipation and restraint allowed Dr. Rho to construct and unleash the sentence that would ultimately lock away my past forever while unlocking a feared and un-wanted future. "Jared has Leber's Hereditary Optic Neuropathy and will soon lose sight in his other eye as well," Dr. Rho said. "I'm so very sorry, but Jared will be blind." I guess Dr. Rho understood that the sounds she then heard were my parents' phones crashing to the floor and my parents sobbing uncontrollably.

Blind, what the hell was blind? I'm eleven years old. I'm a hockey player. I dig chicks and they dig me. I've got a lot of friends and no worries. Blind? What do they mean I won't be able to see? Not be able to see what? What are they telling me? What am I going to be able to do? Who is going to want to be around me? Why me? I thought, "Just fix it, Dad, and let me go play with my buddies."

I guess I would have dropped the phone and cried too if I had truly understood as my parents did the difficulties I would soon face. Instead, my crying came months later when I went blind in my other eye. It was then that I became aware that the exciting life I had once lived and treasured died with my last look at the world. That at the age of twelve, the life I was familiar with could only be experienced in my dreams at night and my nightmares would be experienced during my waking hours.

What ensued from well wishers were comments like, "You've got to make lemons into lemonade," and "You've got to play the hand you were dealt." I especially loved, "What doesn't kill you makes you stronger," and the classic, "When one door closes, another door opens." Sure, it's easy for you to say. The fact is, I missed my true love, hockey, and didn't know how I could live without it. I couldn't imagine a life without the smell of the locker room, or the camaraderie of a team, or the intensity and excitement of the greatest sport on earth.

My seven years of hockey before I lost my sight were probably the one thing that kept me in the game of life. It taught me that through effort, dedication, and focus one could realize success. When I was eleven, our team won the Florida State Championship, which was a miracle when you think about a team coming from Orlando, Florida. Unlike Tampa, who had the NHL Tampa Bay Lightning, and Miami, who had the NHL Miami Panthers, Orlando didn't have an NHL team by which to be mentored. It was the greatest moment of my younger days—winning the Florida State Championship—and was probably one of those events that provided me with the constant need to move forward and succeed.

As I grew older, hockey took a back seat to one of the most fundamental human needs that is often taken for granted, and something I lost and thought I'd never have again: FREEDOM: Freedom to engage those around me; Freedom of movement; Freedom to choose; Freedom from fear; Freedom of no limitations; Freedom from being different; Freedom from dark thoughts; Freedom to cultivate relationships. Freedom is the gate to positive thought, creativity, and prosperity. Would I ever be able to find freedom again?

"Hey Jared," my mother called out. "How about going to Guitar Center and checking out guitars?" What the hell was she talking about? I hated music. Well, I listened to rap, but I never heard guitars playing with rappers so why would I be interested?

"Uh, no thanks mom." I knew she was just trying to get me interested in something that could possibly take the place of hockey and give me something to do, but give me a break. How could a guitar ever give me the same feeling as checking an opponent into the boards and watching them fall to the ice or slamming in a game winning goal? Damn, those were great times. Little did I know then that my mother's ridiculous question would eventually lead me to finding freedom once again.

I can distinctly remember my first visit to Guitar Center and hooking up an electric guitar to an amplifier. I had never seen anyone play a guitar, nor would I ever, and I couldn't think of any songs that had a guitar part so the experience was less than thrilling. I really didn't know why I was there and neither did those listening to the noise that was coming from my amplifier, but getting out of the house was a pleasure. It was that freedom thing. So there I sat making unbearable noise for the better part of an hour. I had nothing else to do so what the hell. I remember my father apologizing to customers and employees for my ear shattering note selections, but everyone showed empathy. Not necessarily for my blindness, but for their recollection of their first time on the guitar.

I really don't know why, but I allowed my parents to buy me a guitar and an amplifier that day. Maybe like a hockey stick, it felt good to hold something in my hands that seemed to have enormous power. Maybe I realized I needed something to fill my days of solitude. Maybe I was just trying to please my parents. Maybe I sensed limitless musical talent and creativity within me that I was going to share with the world. Yea, that was it. Sitting there playing noise on an instrument I had never held or would see, I knew it was my destiny. Right!

I could pull at your heartstrings and say that I lost many friendships when I lost my sight. I could say that, and it would be the truth. However, there is always a flip side to every story. Those I lost were not worth friendship. That may sound too harsh, and it is, so I take it back. I mean, how does one at any age process tragedy and find the strength, time, and appetite to assist those in need? My friends who did stay by my side were totally and unequivocally unbelievable. They provided me the courage and willingness to begin my new life without sight and I didn't want to let them down. They were my cheering section and, well, it goes back to my hockey days when people in the stands would cheer me on. It would just make me skate faster and play tougher. I can still remember my grandfather screaming during my home games, "Get the puck out of there!" We still have a good chuckle about that one.

So you may be wondering, what it's like to be a blind person in a sighted world? Well, the only way of truly understanding another person's life is to walk in their shoes. So, if you can muster up the courage, close your eyes, even if it's just for thirty minutes. Now put your hand on the shoulder of someone you trust and allow them to lead you around a mall, a street, school, or go to a restaurant. Ah ah, no peeking.

After a few minutes of laughing with your human guide dog, you should begin to feel very uncomfortable. Not only about your safety, but about how difficult it is not to see what others are doing or the expressions on others' faces. Not only about how you think others are staring and judging you, but that you cannot experience the visual stimulation that once co-existed with and promoted numerous emotions. As a matter of fact, your strongest emotion now will be fear. Thirty minutes, that's all it takes. You will find that most everything you appreciate in life, the things that make you happy, the moments you treasure with all your heart, have all been experienced with your sense of sight.

Hold on, I know the next question you are thinking. Can a person who is blind truly be happy? I would ask, can anyone truly be happy? Are we not all imprisoned in some form with negative thoughts about ourselves, our shortcomings, our inhibitions, and our fears? Don't we all hide behind a mask of deception so others will accept us, so we will accept ourselves? So my answer is, yes. A person who is blind can present themselves as happy, just as sighted people do. However, like everyone, we hide our sadness and constant struggles even from ourselves, thereby allowing the existence of endless possibilities.

There are endless possibilities. "Jared, there isn't anything in this world you can't do if you put your mind to it," my father would say. Dr. Hakim, a family friend, would share his thoughts: "Jared's spirit for life and success will not die with his vision." Again, it's easy for others to say. I mean, they aren't living in darkness. But, what the hell, maybe they knew something I didn't. So I gave it a shot.

My guitar lessons began at the age of twelve, and like hockey, I dove in with both feet. Though I had no idea where it would take me, I practiced that instrument ten hours a day. I even slept with my guitar, which was always a constant joke around the house. I guess a psychiatrist might say it became my way to escape my sadness. But since I never met a psychiatrist who wasn't more in need of psychotherapy than I was, well, you decide why someone with no love for music and no previous talent for it would immerse themselves in it.

About psychologists, a funny story to share. My mother and father went to one seeking advice after I lost my sight. At the end of the session, they were handing tissues to the doctor as she was talking not about me, but about the problems and sadness in her own life. "Hey doc, what am I, chopped liver?"

One thing about life: we are never smart enough to see the future. We can work hard and prepare ourselves for the future, but we just never know how the game will be played or if it will eventually be won. I guess that's what keeps us moving forward: the hope that things will get better; that we will emerge victorious. Even if there's only one minute left in the game, down by two, your goalie is in the penalty box, your coach has gone home to dinner, and your legs feel like 200 pound weights. You just keep going strong until the buzzer goes off because you never know. You just never know.

So while practicing the guitar, I guess I had hope that it would open up a new, thrilling, uncharted journey for me; and amazingly, it did. As I progressed, I began to feel better about myself and my accomplishments. People were noticing that I was becoming quite good and there's nothing more motivating than others praising you.

One of my favorite bands, "Shinedown," was coming through Orlando to play a concert and my father called them to ask if I could meet them. Well, not only did I get to meet them, but they let me play a song with them onstage in front of seven thousand screaming fans. The feeling I got from that event made me practice harder and study more than I ever thought possible. It made me want to get back onstage as quickly as possible, but next time, I wanted it to be with my own band.

"Sound Cannon" is the name we came up with for our band. It formed around three years after I played with "Shinedown," and we were pretty darn good. After just a year of being together, we were voted the second best band in Central Florida, which was huge because there were bands who had been on the scene many more years than us.

The smell of my clothes after a concert wasn't nearly as bad as was the smell permeating a locker room after a hockey game. But the camaraderie of our band and being onstage playing music to a packed house of adoring fans was just as intense and exciting. It really felt like we were on our way, but then sadly and unexpectedly our singer died, and with him, so did our hopes for the future. We were crushed.

Oh boy, here they come again. "You've got to make lemons into lemonade." "When one door closes, another door opens." I thought, "Crap, I'm seventeen, I can't see, we lost our friend and talented singer, and now we have to start all over again. Is there any chance I could catch a break? Could something go right for a while or does life just keep dumping on you? Are we all tested? Wasn't I tested enough? What did I do to deserve this? What's the point of going on?" Do I sound bitter? Well I was.

After weeks of depression and anger, we began looking for another vocalist. I guess we came to the realization that we didn't want to die with our friend; that we still wanted to live life and bring back those special moments we had once encountered; that bad times were a part of life and just beyond bad times are good times. So we settled on another singer who didn't have the talent or focus we needed, but nevertheless, we took him on an East Coast tour for three weeks before letting him go. It seemed that was it for "Sound Cannon." We were spent and finding a vocalist who was as talented as our first vocalist seemed improbable.

OK, so here it comes again and now, for the first time in my life, it made sense: "When one door closes, another door opens." Maybe I was more mature. Maybe I was ready for a change. Whatever it was, I was all too happy to walk through the next door.

The door to "Sound Cannon" was about to close for a while and I needed a plan, a goal, a reason to continue with music. I was slowly giving up on the idea that I was going to be in a successful band or that music was going to be my life. I was definitely in a funk and I needed some motivation. Two things got me back in the game: Sam Ash Music Stores Guitar Competition and Musicians Institute.

Bryan, my bass player in "Sound Cannon," came to me one day after our band broke up and said, "Hey dude, Sam Ash Music Stores is having a guitar competition and you should enter because the prizes are really cool." Damn, I had nothing going on and to be honest, I think we all wonder how our talents measure up to others'. Everyone had always told me I was good, but I thought they were just being kind because, well, you know; I couldn't see. So I told Bryan to enter me in the competition, which was perfect timing because I needed something to focus on.

Well, to make a long story short, I won the store, city, and regional competitions, which was totally awesome, and I was sent to Los Angeles for the National Championship. OK, so it didn't end up with the Fairy Tale ending: "Blind Guitarist Wins National Guitar Championship." I did feel like a bullet train ran me over when I lost, but life is about perspective. I know that now; I didn't then. I mean, I did win three out of four. I did get to meet my guitar idols who were the judges in Los Angeles, and I guess by making it to the Nationals made me realize that even though I lost, I must have been pretty good to get that far. So when I stopped beating myself up for losing, I felt great about where I was and where I was going, to Musicians Institute.

Back when we were on the East Coast concert tour with our second vocalist, my father said, "Jared, you know when we let our singer and drummer go when we get back to Orlando, you're going to have options. I know we talked about music school before and maybe now is the time that it makes sense for you to go."

I throw the words "on tour" out very loosely. It sounds like we were playing in front of a zillion people every night. The fact is, most nights there were more in our band than in the audience. Sure, there were a few nights we kicked ass in front of large crowds, but when you do college towns in the middle of summer, well, not so smart.

It still was great to travel around and get out of Orlando for three weeks. FREEDOM. While the others were always excited about where we were going and what new sights we would encounter, it was just great for me to be on the road. The act of traveling is fun. Where I go and what sights are there are incidental. It's the feeling of traveling that unlocks some of my happiest moments growing up. I learned at an early age it was the journey that was really fun, not necessarily the destination. Traveling, yea, it's great.

Chicago was the most exciting stop for me on the tour because I was born and raised there until I was four. I was familiar with the city and always had a love for it. There is a certain connection, an unconditional bond, a comfort with places I saw before losing my sight because I still can remember them. It's like running into an old friend. "Hey Chicago, it's great to SEE you again!"

So, you might be wondering about my mother and father. Well, my parents went through hell when I lost my sight and to be honest, I know they still mask their sadness around me. I mean, c'mon, let's be real. How can parents be giddy and gay when their child can't see? What's truly amazing is the therapy they sought out in the beginning. When I say they, I'm really referring to my father. I mean most people would have gone straight to a psychiatrist, a priest, a rabbi, or even a support group for therapy. Not my dad. He dealt with his depression by trying to do "good" for the world. I really didn't get it then and I kind of get it now. But hey, we all have to play our own game, right?

The first thing he did was create a documentary called "Blindsided" that unveiled our families' most intimate thoughts and emotions after I lost my sight. My father wanted to give hope to other families facing their own tragedies. In my opinion it was totally premature because we were still up to our butts in confusion, depression and whatever else you could imagine. I certainly wasn't feeling very hopeful and neither was my mother nor sister Audra. But, it gave my father a distraction and amazingly, "Blindsided" ended up on HBO for two years. If you want to check out an uplifting documentary about how a father destroys his once beloved family, after learning his wife passed on a genetic mutation that made his son blind, and how this young boy (that's me)—through his unbelievable, indomitable, and steadfast courage (probably too many flattering adjectives)—brings his family back together, go to Blindsidedthemovie.com.

Now, one would think that the documentary was enough therapy for my father; that he gave the world something special and it was now time to move on with his life. But he was just getting started. I think he was still trying to make reason out of what happened to me instead of just saying, "Shit happens for no reason."

So now, we were going on to TalkingTabs.

I learned to play the guitar by my teacher telling me where to place my fingers and what strings to play. When my father noticed how well I was doing, he, with the support of my mother who really wasn't comfortable opening up our lives for "Blindsided," decided to start a company called TalkingTabs. This company would teach people who are blind how to play the guitar using verbal instructions on audio CDs.

So he brought in guitar teachers and engineers, and in over five years created the most incredible audio guitar lessons ever developed. The problem lies in that you can probably count on your hands and toes the total number of blind people who want to learn to play the guitar. It's not an easy instrument to play. The piano is much easier and the drums might be the easiest. However, since I played the guitar and he saw how it helped me out of my misery, that's what my father wanted to be taught to other people who were blind.

I think my father sunk most, if not all his money into TalkingTabs, but I truly believe he has no regrets. I heard him laugh a while back with my mother that if all the people who were blind in the United States learned to play guitar using TalkingTabs, he still wouldn't get his investment back. But he didn't do it to make money. He did it to make a difference and to make reason out of what happened to me.

I now think my father is cured and doesn't require any more therapy, which is great because I don't think he can afford any more. As a matter of fact, I know he's cured because I heard him say to someone just the other day, "Shit happens for no reason." It just takes some people a little more time to accept reality.

So here I am at Musicians Institute in Los Angeles, California eight years after playing my first ear-piercing concert for my mother and father in Guitar Center. I believe I'm the first blind student that has attended this remarkable music institution, which is pretty cool. I guess they believed I was good enough to keep up with all the other students who are required to read music. I finished my first quarter with a 4.0, which is a miracle because after the first two weeks, I didn't think I was going to be able to continue.

School is very hard since I have to figure out everything on my own and memorize what everyone else is reading in music books and on the blackboards during classes. But that's OK because while the others are strengthening their reading skills and will be able to play anything put before them, I am strengthening other music skills that they will never attain. It all evens out and in the end; we will all find tremendous fame and fortune. All right, no one can see the outcome of the game. I am just being hopeful.

I wish I could give you an uplifting philosophical ending to this story, but the game still has a lot of time left on the clock and you just never know, right? However, you've come this far with me, thank you, so I'd like to give you the ending to now.

I always hated hearing that number 11778. It snatched the sight right out of me and with it, the life I knew and loved. Yet on the other hand, it unlocked something within me, something that expressed itself, something that was as predisposed in my DNA as my mutation at nucleotide position 11778: a passion for music and an ability to comprehend, memorize, create, and play music at a professional level.

My journey is far from over and even though obstacles abound, I know I'm on the right path. I'm surrounded by amazing music teachers in an incredible music environment situated in the music capital of the world. It's good times now.

After Musicians Institute, where I'm trying to become the best I can be, I may rebuild Sound Cannon, or create music for movies, or tour with another band, or open a recording studio, or may even write songs for other bands. It almost sounds like I've found freedom again, doesn't it? Cool.

Some say I've made lemons into lemonade or I played the hand I was dealt. I say, "You have to keep going strong until the buzzer goes off because you never know how the game will end. You just never know."

Jared Hara

*** Very exciting update on Jared—"Hollywood Music in Media Award for the Best New Rock Song 2012"

http://www.soundcannon.com

http://www.jaredhara.com

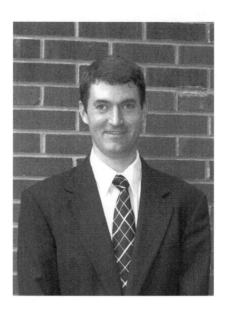

Locke's Story

Old men always seem to dress in a style that's from a bygone era. I have a theory on that. I used to have a different theory. My old theory was that they got stuck in the style they had when they got married. After that, they no longer had to try and impress women. I was wrong.

I realized I was wrong when my wife, girlfriend at the time, affectionately told me I dressed like I was in the 1990's. She actually told me I dressed like Jerry Seinfeld, but she meant the 1990's. She told me that in 2006. We met in 2005, which is a tribute to her politeness. My new theory is old men get stuck in the style from the era when their wives give up trying to keep them looking good. My wife has kept me in style ever since we started dating.

When my wife told me I dressed like I was in the 1990's, one thought went through my head. I dressed like I was in 1993. 1993 was when I could see. 1994 until now is when I could not.

I had spent my life hating school. I didn't hate learning. I am an Eagle Scout. That took some learning: twenty-one merit badges of learning. I loved learning to drive, to play golf, to play pool, and to train my dog. I enjoyed art class, PE, and drafting. I hated the busy work. Why do ten math problems if you learned how after five? A chemistry assignment I had one time required solving formula after formula for about ten pages of solving. They were all the same pattern. I quit after I figured out the pattern. Fool me fifty times, shame on me; fool me 500 times, shame on you.

Needless to say, I was not valedictorian. I originally wanted to be an architect. That was only because special operative for the Phoenix Foundation, otherwise known as being MacGyver, was not a real life job. My dad told me I was going to have to have better grades to get into the school of design. I took this under advisement and promptly decided to be an engineer. My dad told me my grades were going to have to improve if I was going to get into the school of engineering. I took this under advisement and went to the driving range. My dad told me I was going to have to not do any worse if I was going to get into NC State. My guidance counselor took the same position and handed me a curriculum guide. She said to find another major than engineering.

I browsed the catalogue and right after Engineering was Forestry. Ok, so maybe English came between Engineering and Forestry, but MacGyver never disarmed a bomb with a semicolon. The point is, I never even knew Forestry was a major. It is an actual curriculum that includes being outdoors, setting fires, and using chainsaws. I applied immediately.

I started NC State in the fall of 1993. I had a calculus professor who did not give busy work. I had mandatory PE. Introduction to Forestry had more class time outside than inside. I also had biology, in which I promptly got a 60 on the first exam. Never having studied, I did not know how to.

I made a lot of friends quickly because I was confident, funny, and easy-going. It was my first time living away from home, so I bought the 1994 Sports Illustrated Swimsuit calendar. I think I set it to July. It's not like it was even 1994, and I liked July. She was wearing a silver swimsuit and gazing out at the ocean. Yes, that was a beautiful ocean. Things were going great.

Then one day in late September, I woke up and noticed a blurry spot when I looked at the alarm clock. I thought it was a contact lens. Sometimes I slept with them in. Later, walking to class, I still noticed it. It felt like there was some film on my eye. I took my contact lens out. When I got back to my room, I put a new one in. The blurry spot was still there.

I called home. My mom called the eye doctor. She relayed back to me that the doctor said it was probably nothing and to use my glasses for a while; it was probably just optic neurosis. My mom scheduled an eye appointment for fall break.

I took a visual field test. The doctor isolated the blind spot that had formed. He still thought it could be optic neurosis, but wanted to have some other tests and to send me to another doctor, who was a specialist. I had other tests. I had a CAT scan and an MRI. I was diagnosed with severe sinusitis. That turned out to be a cyst on my sphenoid sinus. It is the sinus that runs parallel to the optic nerve and a cyst had put pressure on it. Moreover, the specialist said there is a condition called Leber's Hereditary Optic Neuropathy that he wanted to rule out. He had blood drawn and sent to Iowa. Somewhere in Iowa is where they were testing for the genetic marker in those days.

The test came back positive. I had the Wallace Mutation. It is usually triggered by environmental factors. I was told not to drink or smoke and to avoid exposure to environmental toxins. The disease plateaus out around the six to nine month mark and sometimes improves.

I had minor surgery on my sinus to remove the cyst. It was benign; however, it was likely the environmental trigger. We know of no other.

My fifth grade teacher, my very mean fifth grade teacher, made students bring boxes of tissue to school. She told us she never wanted to hear us sniff. She told us sniffing was bad for our sinuses. We all still sniffed. I haven't sniffed since 1993.

Life did not change immediately. I went back for the spring semester. I had a closed circuit video enlarger. I explained what was going on to my friends. They stood around not knowing what to say like most college boys would do.

I started not being able to follow the writing on the board in classes. Doing homework with a video magnifier was slow. My grades were dropping.

My friends all went on a ski trip. I stayed behind, not being able to see well enough to ski. Things were changing faster than I had thought.

I withdrew for the semester and went home. I had a good friend from high school who was a couple of years younger than me and had not yet graduated. He was glad to have me back in town. I was glad for that.

That summer, when time finally caught up to my Sports Illustrated calendar favorite month, which, at the time, was under my mattress, we took a family vacation to my great uncle's time share at a golf resort. There was not much to do there but play golf. It was going to be a nice break. I had some new clubs that I was hitting solidly on the driving range.

My sister rode with me. She was going to help spot my shots when the ball got out of sight. The first round I lost 10 balls on 10 shots. I could not line my shots up. I hit my last golf ball and lost it like the others. My hands shook as I put the club back in the bag. My golf game ended. When I slid my iron back into the bag after careening my last ball into the woods, it was an instant transition. I went from being in the game to being a spectator; from being a part of the fun to watching other people have fun. It was the longest vacation of my life. Golf was all around me and I couldn't play. I couldn't even enjoy the swimming pool without thinking about how I wasn't playing golf. I was glad when that vacation ended.

Although my vision had significantly worsened, I still had enough sight to walk in the woods. I could head straight out our back yard and walk for more than two miles before coming to a paved road. It was more than that to either side. I would walk during the days. I would take Sydney, my Australian Shepherd, and explore the back yard. Sydney was headstrong and active. She would get into a cow pasture and have 50 cows in a tight group within minutes.

Sydney was also stubborn. We got her when she was a puppy. It was before my vision problems started. She was in a litter of four. One puppy was in the corner sleeping. Two others were fending off the playful assaults of the fourth. My dad said the most active one will be the healthiest. We picked her. I took her for a run through the woods for the first time several weeks later. She was keeping up with my pace. I stepped on and over a large fallen tree leftover from Hurricane Hugo's path. Sydney wasn't behind me anymore. I went back to find her waiting patiently at the tree, determined only to go the way I had. I picked her up and over and we kept going.

One day, before my vision problem started, my sister, Sydney and I were walking. We came to a creek. Sydney got there first and was soaking wet. She was running up and down the creek bed. My sister and I waited and let Sydney run some energy out. She did, and came by us panting hard. Then as dogs do, she shook a gallon of water out of her fur and on to us.

We then started to cross the creek. My sister crossed a small five inch diameter tree that had fallen across some time ago. I crossed next. Sydney tried, and fell into the creek. She tried again, and again, fell into the creek. I went back and came across wading through the water. Sydney followed through the water that time.

I would walk in the woods almost every day after I had withdrawn from college. My friends were in school or working. One day, when I was walking with Sydney exploring new areas, it was getting time to turn around and head home. I turned around, and couldn't tell which way I had come. I couldn't see the path. I walked one direction and hit a briar patch. I redirected and hit more briars. My chest tightened. It wasn't from a fear of being lost. I wasn't lost. I knew where I was. It was from the fear of one more thing. I was losing, my ability to roam the woods. My general sense of direction was intact, but the specifics of avoiding fallen trees, of not stepping into ditches, and of finding a clearing through a briar patch were disappearing.

I knew the direction I needed to go. I looked off at the horizon, at the grey hazy afternoon sky casting shadows onto the tree line at the top of the hill. I thought about the briar patch between me and the tree line and took a deep breath. I headed in. I took high steps, trying to pound down the branches. My arms and legs were getting scratched, but it was my shirt and shorts holding me up, getting stuck to the thorns. I forced my way through.

Sydney followed. She could have easily gone around. She knew the way we came, but she followed me. Then I didn't hear her for a few steps. I turned back. She was stuck in briars. Her fur was caught. Her paws were not even touching the ground. It had to have hurt for her not to keep forcing through. She was determined to stay by my side whatever I was going through.

I picked her up. I had to walk backwards then, to shield Sydney from the briars. They caught my back some, but not my face or arms. It was actually faster, and I pushed on through to the clearing.

Whatever I was going through, whatever I would go through, Sydney was going to stick by my side.

My family was like that too.

When people interact with me, they tend to reveal themselves, whether they want to or not. People who otherwise seem shallow show themselves to be understanding and open. People who seemingly are open and understanding tend to fade out. And then there are the people who try, but cannot understand beyond their own perception.

I found out who my real friends were and what kind of friends I want in my life. When I withdrew from NC State and came back home, Michael welcomed me back and included me in all his adventures. When I went back to NC State, I went back to the same group of people I left. Most included me to an extent, but more and more so, they started doing things without me. Some started out going out of their way to include me, and going overboard with trying to help me. By overboard, I mean handing me a banana and telling me it's a banana type of overboard. These are the people that could not understand beyond their own perceptions. They figured they know it's a banana by seeing that it's a banana and do not understand that I can hold a banana and know it's not a watermelon. One friend, who is still one of my best friends, treated me no differently and seemed to have an intuition of how much to help. In his high school days, he was a geek and so somewhat of an outcast, at least in the view of the cool kid cliques that go on in high school and the first part of college.

When I came back to NC State, I was equipped with some of the latest technology for assisting the vision impaired. I had a Magni-site closed circuit magnifier. I could put papers underneath the camera and have them blown up and displayed on a regular TV. I had a 286 speed processor computer equipped with Word Perfect. I memorized the keystrokes to get into a blank document and then to save it to a disk. I would take the disk to the tutor and she would help revise and edit it. I did not do this too often. It became easier for most papers just to dictate from scratch rather than try to fix all of my typos. Disability services helped provide me with text books on four sided audio cassettes and with note takers in my classes. The bright side of this method of studying was that even though I was learning a completely new way, it wasn't like I was throwing out all these great habits developed throughout the years.

The disability services office provided me with tutors to help me with my assignments. I was provided Mary Rose Raufer. She was in her early seventies at the time. She did not like finding a study room on campus, so I would go to her house. She would pick me up most of the time. I also rode a short bus. It isn't as embarrassing when you can pretend no one is around.

They provided me with a note taker. This is a volunteer from each class who would take their notes on carbon paper and tear off a copy for me. Even though I couldn't read from paper any better than I could read the board, I could have Mary Rose go over the notes with me.

My books came on tape. I had a tape player with an adjustable speed. I listened fast.

I had a reduced course load in order to adjust. I gradually built up to a more normal load. Navigating to class and to the dining hall was harder than the classes, initially.

Disability services offered up their work study employees to help me learn my way around. Fortunately I did have that semester where I could see, and I had explored campus thoroughly. I liked new places. I had a good idea where everything was located. I still needed help with some intersections and locations I had not paid attention to before. There are different sets of details needed with low vision. Noisy air conditioners are more useful landmarks than signs.

I continued in the Forestry program. I knocked out as many of the courses as I could, such as music and other electives, before getting to the more difficult-to-accommodate courses. Dendrology came.

Dendrology is tree identification and study. It is a course where students learn to identify over 200 different species of trees, in the field, and by their fruits, nuts, and cones. That's over 200 to get an A. It's around 165 to pass.

We had a two-hour lecture once a week and then once a week, a four-hour field trip to learn the trees. I threw-up before the first few field trips.

I got a C. I am more proud of that C than any A. Part of the C was due to my continued ignorance in basic biology because I learned the trees. I could touch the trunk and feel around the ground for a leaf or seed, and hang in there with the rest of the class. They did give me a free pass on identifying Poison Ivy by touch. I still had to know the scientific name, Toxicodendrons Radicans of the anachardiacae family.

That was the last Forestry course I could take before the summer camp. It had been more than two years with no significant improvement in my eyesight. Two years was as much of a benchmark for spontaneous recovery time as the doctors could give. I had to finish college blind.

I went with the lead summer camp professor and the disability counselor to the campsite. The camp professor talked about the different courses required: fire management, mapping and mensuration, to name a few. We walked from area to area in the camp site with the professor describing what the students are required to do in each class. There was controlled burning, use of heavy equipment, drawing maps, and measuring large distances and sizes. For every class, the disability counselor would come up with some elaborate way the course could be accommodated for my disability.

We eventually came back to the main area where we had started our tour. The professor, without asking if we minded, pulled out a cigarette, lit it, took a long puff on the cigarette and exhaled, and said, "Well, that's it." The disability counselor coughed more than she needed to and waved off the smoke with her notepad. She answered, "We can find a way to do it."

It should not go unmentioned that I rode out there with the disability counselor and rode back with her. The Forestry summer camp professor drove himself.

It was one of those moments when I think, I have always been healthy. I never smoked. Why does the smoker get to be the forester? Why does the smoker get to see? Why can he take his health for granted without consequences?

The disability counselor was an African-American. I mention it because given her age and being in the South, it can be assumed with 100 percent certainty that she faced prejudice in her life. Sometimes she had to work harder to keep even. She may have coughed more than she needed to, but I don't think she coughed too much. She told me again, "We can find a way."

Maybe we would. Then I could have had the summer camp credits and then find a way to take the other courses, and eventually get my degree in Forestry. But it wasn't like being a history major and having a driving course requirement. It was like having a driving major and a driving course requirement. These were courses necessary for the jobs I would be qualified for with my major.

There are only a few times in my adult life when I cried. That night was one of them. I needed to switch majors. I scheduled an appointment and talked to my advisor. I always enjoyed going to see him. Other students were afraid of him. He was as bald as they come, but if he told someone he had hair, they would tend to agree. What the people who were afraid of him did not realize was that he didn't want you to agree. If you agreed, he would question you to find out why. It was a no nonsense gruffness, not a meanness. If you gave an honest and complete statement, everything went fine.

I told him the disability office is willing to do whatever it takes to provide accommodations for me to take the summer camp. The thing is, it wouldn't be me taking the summer camp, I would be watching the accommodator take the summer camp. And then the accommodator would have the skills I needed to get a job and I would have the skills of being able to describe what the accommodator was doing. As poorly as I stated it here, I probably stated it worse when I was 22. Regardless, he understood.

He had a relative with macular degeneration. He told me there was a place for me in the environmental profession; it was just a matter of finding it.

I switched to Natural Resources, policy and administration, still within the college of Forestry. Most of my credits transferred without a problem. For the rest, my advisor told the college they would transfer. And they agreed.

I was making decent grades. I was still in the college of Forest Resources. I was invited to join the forestry honors fraternity.

The honors frat had their pseudo-hazing. New recruits had to make a paddle and get ten other members to sign it. To make the paddle, we had to paint a small oval piece of wood one color and glue it to the paddle shaped piece of wood, painted a different color. Then we had to stencil the frat Greek letters onto the thing, and finally paste a piece of paper with signature lines on the back.

As far as art projects go, this one rated at about a third grade level. I had high school level art training. I could do this project blindfolded, so I thought. Midway through, one of the senior frat boys came in to observe the newbie's' progress. I do not know who this guy was, so I'll just call him Shithead. Shithead came by and looked over my shoulder. He said, "Do you have broken hands?"

My mom was, is, proud of me for being able to join an honors fraternity. She wanted to keep my paddle. I am not surprised. She has kept every art project I have ever made, even if it was gluing a couple of Popsicle sticks together. The paddle is supposed to symbolize achievement. All I think of is the guy's comment.

I was also asked to join the economics honors fraternity. I am a natural at economics. Their hazing involved eating refreshments at the new inductee meeting. I'm a natural at that kind of hazing.

In the summer of 1998, my father learned about a new computer program named JAWS. It is an acronym for Job Access with Speech. It reads text from a computer screen. It echoes as I type and can read back my Word documents and web pages. He bought it for me and helped me learn computers.

One of my biggest worries had been how I was going to work when I got out of college. I relied on tutors and assistance for almost every part of the coursework. JAWS took this worry away. I could write and correct my own papers. I could conduct my own research. In essence, I could work independently.

I started with version 3.1 on Windows 98. JAWS catches up to Microsoft's newest versions. Microsoft then comes out with new versions of their own software. I am writing this on Windows Vista using JAWS version 10.

I graduated in 1999. I did not want to attend the graduation ceremony. To be honest, I had concerns about walking across the stage, or even off the stage. On the other hand, I did not want to be escorted across the stage. Mom, Dad, and Grandma would not let me not go to graduation. I am glad they persisted. I rehearsed. It was not difficult. It was a memorable event.

Graduating was an accomplishment. It was not an end in itself. I had a college education and was jobless.

I moved back home. I did not have a job and the school liked for you to be enrolled to live in the dorms. I started looking for work. Most entry level vacancies in the environmental field required a driver's license for field work or had other vision related requirements. I applied for everything I could squeeze my qualifications into. For the few jobs I was qualified to apply for, I was rejected.

One day I received a mysterious handwritten letter in the mail. It was unsigned, but with an NC State University mailing address. It said to call a certain person at a certain number and ask about an unlisted job with the state Department of Transportation (DOT). I did. It was for a temporary job with the environmental analysis branch.

I interviewed for the position. They asked if I knew GIS (Geographic Information System). I did not. GIS required graphic interfaces. They asked if I could do field work. I said it depends on what it required, but I would need someone to drive with me. They asked what I planned on being in five years. I answered that Governor would be nice.

I think it was my ambition that got me the job, that or my sense of humor. I actually did not get the job I interviewed for. They created a position for me, producing their new environmental newsletter for the branch. It isn't what I planned on doing when I entered college, but it was a job and it involved the environment.

There is a lot of work involved in starting up a quarterly newsletter. I enjoyed it. There is not as much work involved in maintaining a quarterly newsletter. I asked for additional assignments. They gave me some mitigation tracking work, but all in all, my position was becoming less and less purposeful. I was getting bored and there was not much to do about it except look for other work.

I enjoyed living on my own. I was still relying on my parents for a lot of help. I needed help from somewhere. Even if I could walk to the grocery store, and even if I could carry all the groceries back, I still needed help picking out the groceries. The employees helped some, but when it came to meat, produce, and bread, it was better to have someone for whom speed in collecting the items wasn't the primary selection factor, or worse, getting rid of excess inventory, not that I can say that happened.

Vocational rehab sent a case worker out to help with my independent living skills. I showed her how I had learned to do things and she was impressed. She said some things she would take on to help with future clients. She also said I kept a cleaner house than she did. That is scary. The only help she was able to provide was introducing me to raised dot stickers to identify buttons on a flat surface, like a microwave, instead of the gold stars I was using. The dots stick better, but it does not give me that grade-school self-confidence of having a lot of gold stars stuck on everything.

I lived in an apartment complex right on the bus line. I rarely used the bus for anything except going downtown for work. I still had college friends in the area who liked hanging out. Amazon.com had been invented and online shopping filled in some mobility gaps.

The Internet also provided interaction with the world. Through the Internet, I listened to WNCW 88.7, an eclectic radio station from the western part of the state. It reminded me of home.

One day I browsed through WNCW's sponsors' page. I found a vision therapist. I called her. She said they help people improve their vision through various exercises and holistic treatments. Some of their clients have improved to the point of not needing glasses. She talked with me about my condition. She referred me to her guru in Santa Fe.

I spoke with the Santa Fe vision therapist guru. He said he could definitely help. He mailed me some colored cellophane sheets to place over my eyes for color therapy and a bill for a hundred dollars. He referred me to additional sessions with his local prodigy.

I called the local prodigy. She said she could help, or at least not hurt. She could teach me various exercises and therapies. I scheduled an appointment.

I was reluctant to tell anyone I was going to go see a holistic vision therapist. I needed a ride, though. I called my tutor from NC State, Mary Rose Raufer. She would understand. What I needed her to understand was that even the slimmest of chances was worth taking, especially if there is no chance of worsening. She did. I gave her the name of the person. She knew the person. She was long time family friends with this person. That made me more comfortable.

For about eight months, I went to this vision therapist. It was on a monthly basis. She taught me some tracking exercises and a lot of other general eye muscle movement exercises. It did not regenerate my optic nerve, but I do believe it helped keep my eye muscles coordinated and healthy. I still do some of the exercises.

I was getting stifled living in the apartment. As far as apartments go, it was big, 900 square feet, but I was stifled nonetheless. I could follow sidewalks. I started taking walks. I would branch out farther and farther. This satiated my need to explore and roam.

I would walk farther and farther away from my apartment. When I got to a new intersection, I would watch traffic for a few cycles of the lights. I could see general shapes of cars. I could also hear when they were driving. I could not see the traffic signals or any walk/don't walk signs, but I could understand when it was safe to cross. I crossed big intersections, five and six lanes across. I did not tell my mom the size of the intersections, even though she knew I was walking.

The bus drivers announced major roads they were on, and I had a good understanding of where other things in the area were from when I could see. I occasionally checked Mapquest.com, but I did not trust it to even tell me California was west (It has improved a lot over the years). I had an ultimate goal of where I wanted to go.

I was reading a book at the time, The Education of Little Tree, by Forrest Carter. It is about a little Native American boy who was being raised by his grandparents in the mountains of North Carolina or Tennessee. Social Services came around and took him from his grandparents to raise him in an appropriate Christian environment. That stifled him. He would go sit out under the one big tree at the orphanage. Then one day his Grandfather's friend gave Little Tree the opportunity to escape. He did, and Little Tree went back to the mountains. The animals, plants, even the briers, welcomed Little Tree back home.

My goal was the Schenck Forest. One day, I went out Reedy Creek Road far enough to hit the dirt road. It is a magical feeling to hit dirt road. The smells change suddenly. The air is cleaner. Nature welcomed me from the city. Every weekend I would go to the forest. It had a large dirt road path running through it that I could follow. It was about two miles to get there, so I would rarely end up going more than a mile or two once I was there.

During those days, I would go home every two to three weeks. My parents would come get me, usually my dad. We would listen to Reader's Digest on the way home, but mainly just the jokes. I would bring home my laundry, they would get groceries for me, and I would see my dog. We would spend most of the weekend playing.

I switched my work schedule to have four ten-hour days. It made for early mornings, but the long weekends made up for it. I was growing to hate work.

That is improperly worded. I enjoy working. I was growing to hate my job. It had a significant lack of work for me to do. Then, on top of that, I was sitting in a stuffy sea of cubicles while everyone else in my unit was going out to do field surveys at least once a week. I liked the people I worked with, but time spent with them consisted of listening to them rehash stories of being out in the woods, swamps, creeks, and fields: everything I would rather do than sit in front of a computer.

When I was little, around 7 or 8, I caught bronchitis. Under doctor's orders, I was supposed to stay in for two weeks. I didn't mind the first week. I felt sick. The second week, I felt better, but was still stuck. I would look out the window and watch the other kids play. Everything about me wanted to go out.

I was getting this same feeling at work, but sitting in my cubicle at the DOT listening to field stories wasn't the first time I got that feeling. I got it during my forest measurements course. It was one of the last forestry courses I took. I took it after switching my major. The rest of the students were all in the main forestry program. They talked about needing steel-toed boots and which kinds they were buying. These were the same students who slowed me down in my freshman forestry lab. When the Dean suggested a "shortcut" that some of us should take, these were the same students that looked at him like he was crazy, while I ducked under the brush and trekked through to the front.

The class used a lot of formulas. Lectures were slow, partly because I am good at math, and partly because it was a style of teaching that included writing examples on the board and having the students work through them. While the classmates labored, I would work through deriving the origin of the formula from basic geometry concepts. Then I would get that same feeling again. The feeling, at its baser level is simply, "It's not fair."

The new schedule of three-day weekends allowed me to spend more time with Sydney and to condense my time spent in my cubicle. I felt guilty for being away from her. One Sunday night, my parents let Sydney ride back with us. We unloaded the car. We went out to supper. Then they left, with Sydney in the car. Another two weeks were going to go by without her being with me. I wasn't getting anywhere, especially to a point where I was going to be moving out of that apartment. My throat got tight. My eyes got blurry. The next day, I asked my parents if they wouldn't mind if Sydney came to live with me.

Whether they minded or not, they said they didn't. They helped me get what I would need together, and the next time I went home, I came back with Sydney. I was infinitely happier.

I got up earlier and stayed up later. I had to get up earlier to walk Sydney and stay up later to play with her. I was essentially filling a chair for ten hours a day, so lack of sleep didn't bother me. Sydney slept ten hours a day or so. She was not ready to sleep at 10:00 pm for me to get to sleep on time. It was worth it.

On my three days off, I would take her for as long of walks as I could. She went with me to the Schenck Forest. We would breathe the smells of nature together, just like old times.

When we were at home one weekend, after playing in the back yard, Sydney came back in with a limp. This time we knew what it was: her other knee had blown out. We took her to the vet. They didn't even need to x-ray it. We set her up for a second knee surgery.

She had the surgery back home near Statesville, but came back to Raleigh with me during her recuperation. I would carry her out to the yard to let her do her business and carry her back in. She healed, but not back to her full strength. She wasn't able to walk as far as she had.

She could not go as far as the Schenck Forest. That was OK. I was happy walking as far as she could walk and no more. My apartment complex had a small pond with geese. I would take her to wade in it and chase the geese around a little.

By this time, I was feeling guilty for being gone for the ten hour work day. By the time I added my lunch hour and the commute time, it was a full twelve hours. Sydney was a trooper, but she needed more. I redoubled my job search.

I gave up on trying finding work in my field. Everything required field work experience, knowledge of GIS, or a driver's license. There was always some barrier keeping me from being even qualified enough to apply. I found a communications director position for an environmental organization based in Asheville. I got excited. It was a job involving the environment, it was in Asheville, and it did not require field work experience. I applied quickly. I was rejected.

I found a zookeeper position in Asheboro. I applied. It required an Associate's degree in zoo animal technology or equivalent. I figured a Bachelor's of Science in natural resources was equivalent. They didn't. How much of a degree does it take to throw meat to a lion is a question that baffles me to this day.

Government jobs had a long processing time, months. While my zookeeper application was processing, I was realizing I was likely going to need a Master's degree. I was weighing my options. Most of the degrees my undergraduate schooling qualified me for were only going to buy me a couple of more years before I was back in the same position of needing field work experience. I liked soil science, but a Master's in soil science would still require identifying red soil from grey soil. Grey soil signifies saturation because the iron in the soil hasn't oxidized to give it the red color. I could tell the difference between the sandy soil and the mucky soil by touch. Mucky soil is better for making mud pies and sandy soil is better for making sandcastles, for your information.

I found in the local classifieds a posting for a dog kennel manager position. I figured that even though Sydney didn't like too many other people, she did at least like most other dogs, so I looked into it more. It was in Chapel Hill and had housing provided next door. Then I saw it was only part time. I relayed the prospect to my sister, adding that I could get that job and go to law school at the same time, becoming "Mat Locke."

That was the joke that triggered what is now the rest of my life. Lawyers don't need field work experience. I was good at reading statutes.

In what in hindsight seems about as beneficial as asking your waiter if dessert is a good idea, I asked my parents if they thought I'd be a good lawyer.

With my confidence boosted, I had a new career plan. It was none too soon either, because the rejection letter that came in the mail in the next couple of months would have meant seriously contemplating going back to get my Associate's degree in zoo animal technology, majoring in meat throwing with a minor in shit shoveling, or probably the other way around. Nothing against zookeepers, I'm just still bitter about the rejection.

I signed up for the LSAT, the law school admissions test. It was my first standardized test while vision impaired. I downloaded the sample test and timed myself on it. There are four sections: a reading passage section, two logical reasoning sections, and a logic puzzles section.

The reading section presents a long essay and then has a series of questions, like what is the main theme of this passage, followed by A through E of cryptically worded options, none of which seem correct. The logical reasoning sections present short passages followed by a question that asks something along the lines of, what is the main purpose of this passage, followed by A through E options of cryptically worded arguments that make you go back and see if you're reading the right set of answers for the question you just read. The logical puzzle section presents a long section of statements like Alice sits next to Bob, Charlie cannot sit next to Donna, but must sit next to Elaine, and then asks a question like, if Bob also has to be sitting next to Donna, what movie were they watching?

Luckily, I had worked in government long enough to know not to ask what the test had to do with law school, or being a lawyer. I scored myself and had a decent score for taking it cold. My logic concluded I didn't need to study for the actual test.

Maybe I hadn't needed to, but I had not factored in the reader portion. I had a retired engineer who proctored standardized tests to supplement his income. He was well qualified to look at his watch and say, "Begin," and then sit quietly for two hours before saying, "PENCILS DOWN." I used capital letters like the proctor was shouting because that's how I remembered it was when taking the SATs. This particular proctor didn't have it in him to shout. He also didn't have it in him to read for two hours. He read slowly. He couldn't take my directions to go back to specific sections and he would have to always start back at the beginning. He didn't know how to pronounce fairly common words. I should have canceled my score that day, but I am an eternal optimist.

After I got my score, and after I interpreted the scoring system to my chances of getting into law school, I signed up for the next available test. I signed up in a different city to make sure I got a different reader. I also studied.

I watch <u>Jeopardy</u> about every night. I started watching with a different purpose. Instead of seeing how many clues I got right, I started memorizing which contestant got which clue correct, which ones wrong, and which ones went unanswered. Over the next couple of months, I only memorized one full board. My purpose was to build up my short term memory organization to prepare to be able to answer the logic puzzles without writing anything down. It helped.

I studied for the other sections too. I couldn't afford to have a similar score with a different reader. Everything I was reading was indicating how hard it is to increase your score on a second go at it. I was sure it was the proctor, but I needed to improve the score from any area I could find.

I scored better. My score was good enough to be pretty sure I could get into law school somewhere, and my confidence was enough to be able to quit the DOT nine months before my first semester would start. Besides, the unit was moving to another location. It was going to mean I would have to take a 35 minute bus ride to downtown, and then wait to change to a different bus for a 40-minute ride that would take me to a ten-minute walk to the new office. It would have been a 15-minute drive from my apartment by car.

I packed up my apartment, gave my notice, and left the DOT. I moved back in with my parents. They were considerate enough to let me have the upstairs to myself. It was a good time. I had a career path to look forward to, not just a degree with an open-ended question of, "Then what?"

I had nine months to spend a lot of time with Sydney. I would carry her upstairs with me to go easy on her knees. She would sit in the recliner while I surfed the Internet on a 56k modem.

UNC rejected me faster than my application got to them. Wake Forest respectfully declined my admission. Campbell University accepted me to their law school. I visited the school and liked the feeling I got. I decided I would go there even if the other schools hadn't rejected me. Campbell gave applicants a personal look. They went beyond my grade point average (GPA) and my LSAT scores. They saw potential and determination. For that, I am forever grateful to them.

I had to find a place to live. Campbell, then, was in a town with the city limits posted on both sides of the same sign. There was no traffic light. It had a college and a gas station. It was in really more of a sub-town of the small town of Lillington, which was big enough to have a grocery store and a couple of small restaurants, but not a Wal-Mart. For that, we had to go to the multiple, stoplight town of Dunn.

I was nervous about learning a new town and a new campus. Admittedly, I was more nervous about the new campus. The town barely existed. I think my parents were nervous too.

I had a list of rental properties the school gave me. I narrowed them down to the ones within walking distance of campus. I realized the ones within walking distance didn't say pet friendly. I asked when I called. None were. I expanded my walking distance, but then there was more than the distance to contend with. The community was not pedestrian friendly. There was a four-lane highway cutting through one side of the campus and there were no sidewalks anywhere off campus.

I re-called the original places. I asked again, pleading. Fleas were the issue. I persuaded one house to let me move in with a dog if the existing tenants moved out. They didn't. It was either not go to law school or go without Sydney.

I had to go without Sydney. She was about 13 years old. I knew if I went to three years of law school without her, I would never live with her again. I went to law school. It was the right thing to do, but I still feel guilty.

The campus was harder to learn than NC State. It was designed like a Trivial Pursuit board mixed with Chutes and Ladders. At least the campus was small. My apartment was off campus, but closer to classes than my on-campus dorm at NC State.

I moved in. My parents helped. My mom stayed an extra day to help me get orientated and settled. She walked with me, multiple times, to the law school building where the classes were. She did the same to the dining hall until I was comfortable with being able to find it on my own. We did it a few more times until she was comfortable with me finding it on my own too.

The first two students I met at Campbell were Dale, a Korean graduate student and Yoshi, a Japanese graduate student. They immediately befriended me and welcomed me. I ate with them more often than not. Dale would introduce me to other students. I later found out that his name was actually De-yun. Other students later found out my name was Locke, it wasn't Rock. He understood what it was like to have a barrier to learning.

For the most part, the non-law school students were more welcoming and accepting than the law school students. For the most part, the minority students were more accepting than the regular white students. They accepted me as a minority. They understood what it is like to have an extra barrier in life.

If I had to do law school over again, I would do some things differently. One thing I would do differently is I would have not listened to the professors as much. Professors said they did not care about how much we had memorized; they wanted to know how well we understood and how well we think about legal issues. They said if there was a statute that we needed to know, they would provide it. I wouldn't worry about memorizing the rules of law, because rules of law were not provided on any exam. I also would have taken a course in exam answer writing. If I had known there was a basic simple template for all law school exam answers, I could have learned it early on and improved my first semester grades.

First semester grades end up determining the bulk of a student's total law school GPA. The courses and grading get easier and the students all begin to even out.

I had to make the most of my meager rank. The most prestigious internships go to the top ranked students. The honor of editing for the law review goes to the top-ranked students based on the first semester's grades. The criteria employers look to when hiring law school graduates with no experience are internships and GPAs.

There were a few other factors that I had to plow through. I did not have a book for the criminal law course until about four weeks into the class. I had contacted the other book publishers and requested digital copies that I could read with my text-to-speech synthesizer (JAWS). The person I dealt with, Barbara somebody, kept brushing me off and saying I had to wait in line for them to process everyone's orders, that I did not get my order placed soon enough, that I needed proof of purchase of the book sent to them first, etc., etc., etc., blah, blah, blah, yadda, yadda, yadda. The school was reading the book onto cassette tape and trying to keep up with the homework load. They did pretty well.

One day, the professor said he was going to change the reading assignment from the one listed on the syllabus. We were constantly at threat of being called on to answer questions about the reading assignment in front of the entire class. The fear of looking bad in front of our peers and looking unprepared in front of the professor was supposed to encourage us to prepare. I assume it is also supposed to help our confidence about speaking in front of groups.

I went to the professor after class to let him know I would not be prepared for class the next day and asked not to be called on. He asked why I would not be prepared. I explained the situation with the book. He was shocked. He said it was unacceptable for me not to have the book. He asked me for the contact information I had for the publisher. I had the book in Word Document form within 24 hours. The Professor was Anthony Baker. To aspire to emulate his ability to help others confirmed I had chosen the right career.

I have refused to deal with the publisher TW on anything since that date, including their legal research Internet portal. I subscribe to their competitor, Lexis Nexus.

I recently had the opportunity for some retribution with TW. They sent out an email for a free iPod Shuffle, 3rd generation, if I agreed to watch a demo of new law firm software. I quickly agreed. They quickly redacted, saying the offer was not intended for me, only for larger firms. I quickly replied, too late, offer and acceptance, they are legally bound and obligated to send me an iPod. The bottom line to that is, I can hold a grudge. Satisfying grudges, retribution, seeking justice, the lines are often blurred, but, I digress.

I had some other great professors, faculty, and staff at Campbell. The small campus was welcoming and friendly. It wasn't a hundred percent that way, but I won't mention any other names . . . until a little bit later.

I did have an additional barrier, but getting books for following semesters was easier. I did not have good access to some of the supplements everyone else got. Other students used supplements that focused on the essentials of each subject of law. They could trade them around and share them. I did not realize they existed for a while. Then I tried one for business entities class and I was able to just use the supplement instead of the book . . . and instead of listening to the professor.

I signed up for the joint MBA. An Iranian man was Dean at the time. A lecture from him was better than stand-up comedy. Of course, they had him recruiting law students into the MBA program. The MBA coursework was not difficult. I took every advantage of finding the least difficult coursework.

We had the opportunity to take a three week study abroad trip to China through a joint effort with Fayetteville State University. I signed up. I was nervous. Campbell was really the first place I went to where I had to learn new territory on my own. Another law student was thinking of signing up. I had a handshake agreement with her that we would both go. I did not intend on relying on her, but I did want someone in the same hemisphere to know where I was and that I had vision impairment.

The Dean ended up going with us. It turns out it was his brother who worked at Fayetteville State University who helped organize the trip. It was the trip of a lifetime. It was the first time I had gone on a trip of that magnitude without close friends or family. The other students and the professors welcomed me. I often felt like a burden to them, but they never gave any indication that that was the case.

I had a hard time finding an internship. I believe having a disability was a part of why it was hard. My class rank was a bigger part. I interviewed with the Law Offices of F. Bryan Brice, Jr., with F. Bryan Brice, Jr. himself conducting the interview. He formerly worked for the NC DOT, like me. He gave me a chance. I took it.

The internship was in Raleigh. I moved in with my old friend, old roommate, and old DOT coworker. I commuted with him. I had a great summer internship experience. The first case I worked on won and was appealed by the other side. Some research I conducted made it into the opinion. More importantly, during that summer internship, I started dating the woman who became my wife.

Dating is hard when you cannot drive, when you need to ask for help to find the bathroom, when you cannot read dinner menus, and when if you walk your date to the door, you need help walking back. I am lucky. My now wife looked beyond all that immediately. I never felt those concerns when with her.

Having a direction in life helped me get to that initial date with her. It was probably more helpful having the direction than being at the directed point. The direction for me was to become a lawyer. The directed point is being a lawyer. Becoming a lawyer has a sense of justice and nobility that is vastly different than what lawyers end up doing in order to pay the bills. But I digress. Blindness is a part of me, but there is also a wife, family, a career, helping others, etc.

I represented a mother in a custody trial. The grandparents were trying to take custody. They had money on their side and, unfortunately, better facts. They also had the father on their side. Between the grandparents and the father, they had two of the toughest most cutthroat family law attorneys in the area. Every one of their witnesses got two friendly examinations to my one cross. Every one of my witnesses got cross examined twice. The trial lasted an entire week. At the end, my client did not get what she wanted, but the grandparents did not get everything they wanted. It was worth going to trial.

It was a tiring week. At the end, I came back to my office building. I got on the elevator with another couple. I felt the raised numbers for my floor. I pushed the button. One of them congratulated me on how well I did pushing the button.

I spent about a year signed up to a blind lawyers' list serve. I would read posts by blind law students and blind lawyers. I occasionally got some good information. More often than not, I got the sense of over-advocacy.

As a lawyer, we are obligated to zealously advocate for our clients. It is hard to quantify legal requirements stated in ways like, be a zealous advocate. I translate this to mean, on a scale of 1-10, advocate at a level 9. For all the potential clients saying why not a 10, I'll explain. Advocating at a level 9 means that when the other side fails to meet a filing deadline, call the other guy up and ask why they haven't filed; or, if an honest mistake is made, allow them the opportunity to correct it. This should be so because nobody's perfect and that includes you. I will occasionally make a mistake or maybe some time in my career I may miss a deadline. If that happens, I will appreciate the other side advocating at a level 9, and so will my client. Cases should be won or lost on the merits, not on technicalities.

The blind law group over-advocates. On a scale of 1-10, they advocate at an 11. This can put them in a position of shunning things that could help, purely because it is additional help. The help they do accept then becomes an entitlement.

It also seems they want to diminish the value of vision. I think this is because they have often times been blind since birth. Blindness is a part of their identity. Maybe they are also afraid of their ability to participate with sight when they are comfortable with their abilities without sight.

I quit the blind lawyers' list serve. I found an Internet group just for people affected by Leber's Hereditary Optic Neuropathy. It is a forum for people similarly situated facing similar futures. When I was first affected, the Internet did not exist. I had radio, TV, books on tape, and what people told me. It was the Dark Ages compared to today.

The thing about going blind in the late teens, or early twenties, is that to a large extent identity is already on track. We are formulating who we will be. Then we go blind and the proverbial rug is pulled out from under us. We lose everything our identity has been based on.

It bothered me 15 years ago when I was asked if I needed help cutting meat, or knowing I would need help finding a bathroom. I have since married an intelligent and beautiful woman, and I am a solo practitioner lawyer. If someone who knows nothing about me other than what they observe in an elevator congratulates me on my ability to push a button, I will say thank you. My identity is more than blindness. Blindness is something I live with. I am much more than it. I will, however, never accept it. I will never forget what it is like to see. I will do everything I can to encourage my vision to return. I will do everything I can to see again. And, I appreciate all the help people generously provide.

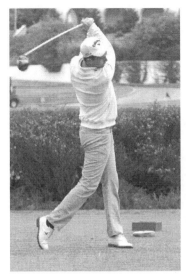
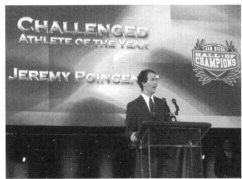

Blindness Won't be his Handicap

When I was diagnosed with Leber's Hereditary Optic Neuropathy I was a college sophomore, thoroughly enjoying my experience at San Diego State University. I was living in a fraternity house surrounded by phenomenal people, at a wonderful campus, in a stunningly beautiful city. I had everything going for me.

I've had 20/20 vision all my life, so you can imagine how foreign it felt for me in the fall of 2008 when for the very first time I had to squint to read something. I remember walking to class one day seeing words on signs, and having trouble distinguishing some of the letters through a very faint blur. This had never happened to me before, so I asked my mom to schedule an optometrist appointment when I was home for Thanksgiving. I figured I was one of the millions of people with below-average vision who need contacts or glasses. Unfortunately that was not the case.

I went to the optometrist the day before Thanksgiving, thinking it was going to be a standard visit. My younger brother came along to keep me company. I could see everything just fine until I was told to cover my left eye. I couldn't see anything on the eye chart, not even the big E. Everything was blurry in the middle. I turned to my brother and said, "Ahhh who needs a right eye?" My mom joined us, thinking we would simply discuss the tradeoffs between contacts and glasses. When instead the optometrist said that the vision in my right eye was worse than 20/400 which was likely due to a pituitary adenoma or a brain tumor, I realized this was nowhere near an ordinary visit.

Most people spend their Thanksgivings gathered around a family table, offering the traditional reasons why they are thankful. I spent the morning in the Emergency Room having an MRI to see if I had a brain tumor. As my family gathered for our feast and tried to act as though everything was normal, I was thankful the test had shown I did not have a brain tumor. My grandfather had died from a brain tumor four years previously, so it was definitely a relief to have that ruled out. But the situation was still extremely frightening, since the doctors weren't sure what was going on.

The next day I saw a neurologist who thought I had optic neuritis, which is basically an inflammation of the optic nerve. This would have been awesome because he said that with a simple steroid treatment for a few days, everything would soon go back to normal. A medical technician came to the house and reassured me that the catheter wouldn't hurt; it only hurts when they have to put it in your hand. He stabbed my arm several times trying to find a vein, but he was unsuccessful. So he switched arms, tried a few more times, and was still unsuccessful. He told me he was sorry, but he had to put the catheter in my hand.

I tried to quell the rumors that were floating around among my fraternity brothers and friends, nonsense spreading that I was totally blind. I told them it was temporary and that I was going to be ok. But I could hear their comments of "Dude, Jeremy's totally blind!" reverberating in my brain as I waited for the vision in my right eye to return.

Unfortunately, my right eye didn't improve. To make things worse, the vision in my left eye started to get blurry also. On the day before Thanksgiving it was 20/30. A week later it was 20/40. Two weeks later it was 20/150. I had to give up driving. As a young adult that's a huge blow to your independence.

Since the second eye doesn't usually lose vision with optic neuritis, the neurologist ordered a lumbar puncture, or spinal tap, to figure out what was wrong with me. For this test they try to numb your back so you don't feel pain. What you do feel is the needle progressively inching further and further into the depths of your spine. Afterwards they put me in a wheelchair and rolled me to a hospital bed.

While I was having that procedure done, my mom was arguing with my neurologist. She'd done a lot of research on the Internet, and thought my symptoms of sudden, painless central vision loss first in one eye, followed weeks later by the second eye, matched what she'd read about a rare genetic disorder called LHON. Since it's passed on the maternal bloodline, she'd called her deceased mom's only living relative and asked if he recalled any stories of blind family members. She was shocked when he replied, "You mean, like my dad?"

Turns out that before my mom had even been born, my grandmother's uncle had suddenly gone blind, was diagnosed with tobacco amblyopia, stopped smoking, and regained his vision a year later, so she'd never known it had happened. Given this maternal family history plus the fact that I was a 19-year-old male, typical for LHON vision loss, she was convinced that's what I had. She printed out lots of information about it to show the neurologist during my spinal tap, but he didn't believe her, told her she was wrong and said that it was Neuromyelitis Optica (NMO).

I didn't know about their conversation, I was just lying uncomfortably in a hospital bed after being repeatedly poked and prodded with needles everywhere. I saw my doctor on my left and my mom on the right. The doctor looked at me and said, "Okay Jeremy, you have one of two things. I think you have something called Neuromyelitis Optica, which will cause you to go completely blind and if we don't treat you quickly you might become a paraplegic. Your mother thinks you have Leber's Hereditary Optic Neuropathy, or LHON, and if she's right you'll become completely blind, you'll have to drop out of San Diego State for 6 months to learn Braille, and you'll need to walk with a white cane or a guide dog."

I've heard of win-win situations, but this sounded like lose-lose. This was not even a month after my initial optometrist visit when I'd thought all I needed was glasses or contacts. Every morning since then I had woken up feeling like my life was a nightmare; now things were getting even worse.

The neurologist asked what I wanted to do. I asked which one might get my vision to return? He said if we treated immediately for NMO I might get my sight back, but if it was LHON there was no treatment or cure. He described the plasmapheresis treatment for NMO as simple; I'd just need a catheter. I figured that was no big deal as I'd just done that, so I told him I wanted to be treated for NMO since it was the only way I might get my vision back.

Only when they started prepping me for the first treatment did I realize that this catheter would be in my jugular vein! So for 10 days I had three cords hanging out of my neck, and every other day I lay in a hospital bed, watching my blood separated and my plasma replaced with synthetic plasma. I remember watching red flow in and out of my neck for four hours at a time.

I was pissed at the world. Why me? Why did I deserve something like this?

I completed five of the seven scheduled treatments before my mom's persistent efforts to get the doctors to locate the spinal tap results finally paid off. I did not have NMO. It was the day after Christmas, and the weirdest sensation was not the broken promise of a cure, but the gasping for air sensation as the catheter was being pulled out of my neck.

In the span of two short months my vision had degenerated from 20/20 to legally blind. I stopped driving. I could not read. I could no longer recognize and distinguish faces.

I was depressed. I was devastated. And I could not forget that if I had LHON, it had no cure. I could not fathom that there were incurable diseases. Except for cancer and AIDS, I thought everything had a cure. I don't know if it was denial, ignorance or something else. The floor of my world had been ripped from under me. I was mean to my parents. I wasn't fun to be around. All I could do was mope around the house.

My mom got me an appointment with the head of Genetics at the Jules Stein Eye Institute at UCLA. She gave him a 100-page document with notes from every doctor appointment I had had since the medical mystery tour had begun, with copies of all my test results. The doctor told me it was the first time he'd ever had a 100-page file on a new patient. He asked my mom if she was a physician and she said no, just a mom fighting for her child.

In his 25 years of practice he had only seen five patients with LHON, but he suspected my mom was right and had blood drawn for a genetic test and told me they'd call me with the results in a few weeks. While I was discouraged to hear that I likely had this disease with no treatment and no cure, he did pick up my spirits by telling me about some of the positive things I could do to overcome my lack of sight. He told me that he had seen hundreds of patients lose vision, and how it would impact my life depended totally on me. He knew some people with only a small loss of vision who let it ruin their lives, and he knew lots of completely blind people that had found ways to do incredible things. He told me, "It's solely up to you to be as successful as you want to be. You can do whatever the "F" you want to do." This was something that I needed to hear, and I took it to heart.

Two weeks later we saw a neuro-ophthalmologist at UCSD's Shiley Eye Center to get a Visual Field Test done. He agreed I likely had LHON, but since he'd only seen one family with LHON in his 35-year career he couldn't answer many of our questions. My mom had seen a neuro-ophthalmology textbook on the Internet authored by this doctor, and it upset her that she knew more about LHON than he and the UCLA doctor did. She searched for a LHON expert, and found that most of the articles about LHON listed Alfredo Sadun as an author. When she realized he was based out of USC at the Doheny Eye Institute, in Los Angeles, not too far from our home, she was literally jumping up and down with excitement.

We saw Dr. Sadun on January 13, 2009. He had answers to all of my mom's questions about LHON. She was the happiest woman in the world, knowing she could finally resign her job as my physician, stop searching for answers to medical questions, and could go back to just being my mom and helping me deal with all the other issues that come along with sudden vision loss. Alfredo Sadun was the first doctor who thought I had LHON that said he wanted to follow up on me. We set up a schedule where I would re-check with him every three months to monitor my vision. He provided me hope. He let me know someone still cared. I was ready to give up on school, on a lot of things. But I found hope in him because he was searching for a cure. It was a great day.

A few days later, on January 16, 2009, the genetic counselor from UCLA called to tell me that the blood test confirmed I had the LHON 11778 mutation. She explained that this was the most common of the LHON mutations, and it had the least likely chance for spontaneous recovery. Some mutations have a 50% chance of recovery, one mutation has 20%, and mine has a 4% chance of recovery.

Since having this experience, I have realized that things can always be worse. When I was fully sighted I took everything for granted. I didn't appreciate the things I have nearly as much as I do now. After losing my sight I realized that I shouldn't take things for granted because in a blink of an eye, they could suddenly be gone.

I've learned that attitude is everything. We all face obstacles both big and small, and it doesn't matter if you're rich or poor, whatever your background, your ability to overcome hardship begins with your attitude. It's how you handle yourself in the toughest of situations that determines your happiness. If you go in with a pessimistic attitude you will never be happy. I think about when you're a kid your birthday is awesome, and I find myself believing that it's because you say that today is going to be a great day.

You have to go in to every day saying it's going to be a great day. Take a deep breath, and will yourself to believe that no matter what, today will be a great day. My biggest thing is attitude. It doesn't matter what you go through, if you're optimistic things will be better, it will always be better. Too many people take everything they have for granted and are unappreciative of the many gifts in their lives. If only they just looked around and paid attention to the people around them and smiled, we would all be better.

It's weird that things like losing your sight have this sort of effect on a person, because normal life gets so routine, and believe me I was immersed in such a routine. At the end of everything, yeah sure, I can be angry that certain things didn't go my way. But instead I've learned to love where I am in life. I've had many great experiences since losing my vision. I've taken up blind golf, and won the 2010 World Blind Golf Championships. I've been featured on several television shows, and have become an inspirational speaker. I enjoy sharing my story because I find that everyone is facing challenges in life and through sharing my experiences, others realize they can get through their own challenges. I am actually thankful for losing my sight because I have become closer to my friends and my family. I've realized what's important in life, and I focus on the positive.

Jeremy Poincenot

www.JeremyPoincenot.com

http://www.lhon.org/lhon/LHON.html

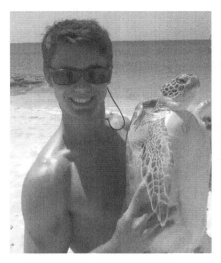
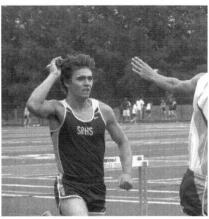

The "Control"

They always say that the hardest part of doing something is starting. Whether it's some work-out program you haven't touched, a new instrument, or in my case, this story, starting is one of the hardest things for me to do. So, let me begin this by saying that I love freeze tag. Freeze tag was something I played on a daily basis during recess in elementary school, and I will always remember the joy involved in that game. However, freeze tag seemed to have its own little passion for me. This very game that I enjoyed so much altered the way I see the world . . . well more accurately speaking it was a metal pole that did the altering, but freeze tag is the very game that led to this story. At the age of six, this is where my journey begins.

It was my first year of real school; I was out of pre-k and was now a "big" kindergartener. I had a newfound liking for baseball, but that all changed in a matter of seconds. A game of freeze tag after one baseball practice started it all. What was once a bright green field with a pavilion to my left and trees off in the distant to either side of me suddenly became a much darker, smaller field with small points where I was able to sort-of distinguish different objects.

William was on the mulch pile, and he was "it." Joey and I were looking back at William running wildly through the playground away from him.

Moving as quickly I could, I hear Joey scream something beside me. I take my eyes away from William while screaming, "What?!" back to Joey. "DUCK!" he screams in return. Now, this is not a duck that goes quack. No, in fact, I turn around and am not greeted by a feathery friend at all. As I turn to see what's ahead, I am greeted by a hard metal pole, right in my eye. That moment, laying there on the ground with a throbbing pain, marked the beginning of a confusing, doctor-filled childhood for me.

I cannot complain about the incident that happened, because in fact, it was probably the best thing that could have ever happened to me at that young age. When you're six, everything is cool. The swollen black, purple, and red eye I received was flaunted and shown off to my class, all of them asking how I got it and if I cried (yes, I did indeed sob). But as that eye became a lighter shade of black, purple, and red my world began to become a darker shade. Over the next year, my eye sight began to get worse and worse until the point that in my first grade year I was legally blind.

Here is just a short paragraph about me. My name is Chase Rudisill and I am a junior at South River High School. I have a younger sister named Jacqui, a younger brother named Grant, an older half-sister named Kristen, dogs, lizards guinea pigs, and a cat. I am visually impaired by Leber's Hereditary Optical Neuropathy (LHON). I have an uncle named Larry, whom is blind. My uncle and my brother are the only other two in my family affected by LHON today. So, let's go back to the incident.

It was an extremely difficult time for my family. Spending quite possibly thousands if not tens of thousands of dollars just on attempts to try and recover my eyesight (I was never told the true amount of money spent). My parents, grandparents, uncles and aunts—nobody knew what would happen or what was to happen, always asking what was to come. My mother was constantly in tears while my father had grave looks on his face. A time of great sorrow for my parents especially; however, what was my opinion of this situation? My face said it all: an enormous, goofy, quite toothless grin stretching from ear to ear.

I was quite possibly the happiest I could ever be: Disney World, airplane flights, doctor visits, hospital Danishes, late night diner waffles, friends galore, Yu-Gi-Oh cards, Pokémon cards, flipping BINOCULARS for school, excitement, and ATTENTION. Primarily a young first grader wants attention, and the fact that I had a "glass eye" and needed binoculars while sitting in the front row too was all I could have ever wanted. Obviously, I did not have a glass eye, but that didn't stop me from telling everyone I had one.

Oh, and "the machine"—a super cool looking reading contraption where a paper or book would be placed under a camera, and from there, the image would be displayed on a computer screen. You could magnify, change colors, and perform many other neat tricks on the text (mostly we put our hands and faces underneath it, though). That reading contraption was my biggest claim to fame. Running into that pole was purely magnificent. I mean, if I got to go to Disney World just for face-planting into a pole, I'd do it much more often. But what I never knew could happen, did happen.

Baseball became impossible to play. The sport I had begun to love to play was now completely gone. All the attention and excitement began to die down, and long distance doctors' visits lost the same cool vibe they initially held. But even worse, it became darn near impossible to go out and run around with friends and play video games. What my parents feared would happen, happened. No more sports. No more regular eyesight. No more normal life.

By this time, I was well into learning how to touch type and read Braille as a safety measure, which especially sucked because I was in the FIRST grade. I already could barely spell, read, or write, let alone learn how to read with dots or memorize finger movements to spell out words I could not even spell to begin with. But I liked my teacher. Actually, I seemed to have much fortune with having "cool" adults around me. I mean, heck, my eye doctor was a magician by hobby. Not many people get some funky eye drops and bright lights shined in their eyes only to discover that somehow, there was a quarter behind their ear the whole dang time.

Also, my uncle, who had gone blind just a few years earlier than me at the age of 19, was a musician, always picking up any instrument around and playing music that I would gawk at. And my touch typing teacher was the nicest person on earth. I went to a small private school where the teachers were all nice to me, and I was also very popular among the parents of most of my friends—I was just that shy, sheltered, blind kid who wouldn't dare go against the rules. Yet, despite all this, some things I did still annoyed some people, especially my friends.

I consider myself a very fortunate individual to not have died of some form of cancer by now—I received a ridiculous amount of radiation from the TV when I was younger, without a doubt. TVs with far away couches were my absolute arch enemy. I loathed them with a passion. I would rather stand up on my own two feet for hours just to watch TV closer than sit on that god awful far away couch. The only problem was if anyone else was watching TV, they would need to stand beside me or else they would see a whole lot of the back of my head and not a lot of whatever we were watching. This got on the nerves of many of my friends.

Anyway, my inability to play outdoor sports and activities caused me to love video games, because in video games I could get as close to the screen as I wanted. It amazes me that playing games 4 inches from the TV didn't kill me, but it sure did a good job at annoying the heck out of my friends.

One morning I was playing a video game called Wario World with my friends, and as I stood about 4 inches from the TV, squinting and trying to utilize what little areas of clear sight I had to see the game, my friends mimicked me and laughed. They poked fun at me by putting their noses all over the TV and squinting as they played. If you've ever put your face ON a TV screen, you'd know you cannot see a darn thing on the TV. The embarrassment was so traumatizing that I decided to move back to about 8 inches from the TV. I know, not much of a difference, but the TV was at least not as bad as computer screens or small handheld devices, those were impossible to see at any distance.

The mother of all things terrible and torturous was the dictionary. My GOD, learning how to use a stupid dictionary was absolutely just . . . horrible. Unless you have had a similar situation to me, you have no idea. Oh, and I have a special message for Where's Waldo: Where the #$%& are you?!

To top my dictionary experiences off, in second grade there were "dictionary races," where the assignment was to find a given word quicker than anyone in the class. I *loathed* those. I was legally blind and there was no way on earth that I was going to be able to quickly skim around a page to find a word on it. I had to take my jolly good old time just slowly staring, one word at a time, finally screaming, "I found it!!" when they had already gone through three more words. That was just an embarrassment to me.

Fortunately for me, my period of being legally blind did not last for a prolonged period of time. With LHON, it is predicted for lost sight to slightly recover, although often this does not happen. Nobody is certain as to the real reason why, but my eyesight recovered remarkably better than was expected. Many factors—my young age, my gene marker (1 4 4 8 4, which is known to be the least severe of the 3 markers), and who knows what else—may have played a role in the large improvement in sight. First and second grade were tough for me, but when I was 8 or 9 and in the third grade, my sight improved dramatically. However, despite the large improvement, there was, and is, still something very wrong with my eyes, and I still can never find Waldo anywhere.

A glorious time for both my parents and me laid ahead, my sight recovered to the point that I signed up for soccer. Soccer had a nice, big, white ball that stayed at a slow, third grade pace and was something I could actually play. In first grade, when I could not see, I had signed up for soccer once. I didn't make it past the first day, having had quite an experience dribbling through cones. The first one third of the cones I turned over; the rest survived only because I went in the wrong direction, not even bringing the ball with me. The ball was lost the moment it exited my small area of visual acuity and entered a cloud of no sight, and the cones were never even seen in the first place. It was incredibly embarrassing, and I was quite the emotional kid. So soccer ended immediately, thought to never happen again.

That first year with improved sight, though, I played division 4 county soccer—the lowest division possible, where we came in dead last. We were absolutely horrible, a record of 0 wins, 0 ties, and all losses (ouch). But there was something about this newfound game that struck me. I was immediately hooked on soccer, and after my first, grueling season, I had the ridiculous goal of becoming a pro.

The ability to play sports was possibly the greatest of all the benefits to gaining much of my sight back. Among the other benefits was the fact that I could play video games from a further distance. I still could not—and cannot—sit on the couch far away and play easily, but my face was no longer practically on the screen. No more binoculars were needed either, thank God, and things were just overall much easier. The weird thing was that my eyesight improved to the point where I could lead almost a totally normal life. Baseball is still totally out of the question, along with other sports such as lacrosse that play with a smaller ball. I don't really feel like getting nailed with a baseball I'm supposed to catch, but cannot see. Soccer, however, became my sport.

Motivation suddenly overcame me in many ways. For instance, I became almost too cognizant about what I ate. It's funny actually, when I was ten I was referred to as a "health nut." Amazing right? A ten year old ACTUALLY concerned about his health. I was more concerned about what I ate back when I was 10 and 11 playing county soccer than I am today at 16 playing high school varsity sports. If it had a nutrition label I was studying that label long and hard. As a ten year old, I made whoever's job it is to write those labels very important jobs, at least to me.

If there is anything I remember about 4th and 5th grade, though, it was my visual field tests. Fifth grade (when I was 11) was the peak of my eyesight, and I am very suspicious it was because I ate much better than ever before. My eyes have never been as good as they were back then, but that's only based off of scientific tests. I have no idea the actual difference because I cannot flip back and forth between 11 years old and present day, obviously. The difference is not large, however it is noticeable. So, what ARE my eyes like?

"Righty tighty, lefty loosey." This same saying for how screws are used can also be applicable to my eyes. My right eye has a very tight world: it is my bad eye, where I have a considerably larger amount of blind spots than my left eye. My left eye, on the other hand, has a loose, open world, for it is far better than my right eye; in fact, my left eye has almost the same visual fields as a normal eye. My nearly normal left eye allows me to compare the difference between normal vision and the effects of LHON. The best comparison I have is this: it's like squinting your eyes, allowing your eyelashes to get in the way of your vision. Now, that is similar to what it looks like, yet it is nowhere near actuality. In actuality, everything is much darker, maybe because not as much light enters my eye, and it is just plain DIFFICULT to see.

For me, there are no clear areas lacking vision I can simply point out. However, it is basically as if too many dots and blobs of all kinds decided to get in the way of my vision to make it hard to see. Don't think polka dots PLEASE. Too many people say, "So it's like polka dots in your eyes! Right?" NO. Not at all. It's more like a foggy window where someone completely failed at trying to wipe off the fog—random areas of no fog where you can see, with some areas of just small tiny spots of fog, with other larger areas of fog where you cannot see. Some with LHON say it is like the TV show Cops, where they blur out the faces of criminals, and I completely agree. When something does happen to go out of sight, it just vanishes as if it were completely blurred out to unexplainable, colorless, shapeless nothingness.

It turns out that in my left eye (my good eye), I only have 52 percent of my optic nerve still living. In my right eye (bad eye), I only have 48 percent. My first thought was, "Why are these two numbers so close to each other, yet the sight is so far apart?" The answer is probably just the placement of the dead nerves. Much of my nerve must have been killed in my original loss of vision; however, in my left eye, the placement of all that dead nerve was so fortunate I am almost unaffected. For my right eye, however, that is not the case.

So here's a little something neat: people have one dominant eye which is used for focusing on objects, while having one non-dominant eye used to allow us to have depth perception and see in 3D. Determining this is simple: Extend both of your hands at arm's length, bring them together to make a small, quarter-sized hole, focus on an object in the distance through that opening with both eyes open first, and then close one eye. If the object in the distance is still visible through the opening, that is your dominant eye. If it is not, that is your non-dominant eye. For me, my dominant eye is obviously my left eye, because I can see best out of it. However, my right eye does not fulfill the job of a non-dominant eye—it does not give me 3D vision.

I've failed every 3D vision test given to me, meaning that basically what I see is, in a way, similar to a movie: a moving picture. I never knew I could not see in 3D until a test about 3 years ago, and the way I have compensated for the lack of 3D is through identifying the size change in objects, not through them popping out from the background and clearly getting closer.

One last thing about my eyes is my contact prescription. If you have contacts or glasses, you would know that the prescription in one eye is very close to, and if not matches the prescription in your other eye. However, mine do not, and this is because of my left eye being so much better than my right. With my left eye, I focus, read, and use it for everything because it is generally much clearer. My prescription in my left eye is—4.50, and in my right—2.50. Usually, the difference between these two numbers is only around 0.25 to 0.50, but mine is 2.0. It is clear that I hardly use my right eye for much of anything.

With everything that LHON has done to my eyes, I consider myself extremely fortunate to have the eyesight that I have. My current vision is the only sight I have any memory of, and I honestly do not mind it; it is a part of me. My sight makes for some pretty great stories too. I thought my baby brother was a dog in the yard one day. I kept asking why there was a dog in our yard, but nope, just a child, false alarm. And one night, as I sat admiring an exquisite mural painted on the side of a Pep Boy's building, I sounded like a blabbering idiot. I was astonished at the detail they were able to get in the various plants and ivy they painted, raving over the skill it must have taken. But it turns out it was just that—real plants and ivy. And there's always the classic: a confused friend because they always wave to you but you "pretend" you don't see them (Sorry dude, you were sort of invisible). Unfortunately, though, I don't tell many people about my sight. I'm not big on dealing with all the questions that come with it.

Things people say to me I find absolutely hilarious: "Dude, yeah, having bad eyes sucks, I know what you mean!" No, no you don't. "Oh yeah, I think I have that too because sometimes I don't see people either," Again, nope. "Wait, so do I have like . . . half a face to you?" Yes. My blind spot makes your face look like a crescent moon (not really). "So when are you gonna get glasses to fix your eyes?" Inform me of the date when you are able to comprehend the word 'incurable' please.

I will give some people credit though, they don't know at all what LHON is, so one or two questions I perceive as stupid is just fine. However, if the stories of how bad their eyes are or about some great eye doctors they get their glasses from continue after I explain further, that's the line. Questions are totally fine, in fact, I love questions. I favor people who I only have to tell once, may ask questions, understand, and life just goes on. However those who wave fingers in my face weeks later and still tell me the wonders of glasses, not so much.

All throughout elementary school I didn't care about telling anyone about my eyes, but as middle school came around I began to think differently about that matter. I went to a small private school for my entire elementary school experience, but in middle school I transferred to a public school. My class size was increased by a factor of about 12. Whereas there were around 30 kids in a whole grade for elementary school, now there were around 350 per grade. Of course I was a little nervous, going into a huge school with practically no one I would know. And a big reason why I didn't tell many people was a result of funny looks from those whom I told. It was as if they said, "Yeah, right, you're just looking for attention." Ironic, because that is all I got in elementary school.

I was a little offended, but I learned quickly not to tell anyone. And still to this day I don't tell people about my eyes unless an event happens where I am forced to tell. Other than that, teachers are the only ones who really know about my eyes, and I am very dismissive when any discussions about placement of my seat or tests arise around other students.

In shorter words, I do not want people thinking of me differently or gossiping about my eyes. I know it is silly to hide, but I don't want a reputation anymore. I would rather have a reputation about sports or academics, not "That's the blind kid over there!" (Especially because I am not really blind, I am just visually compromised.) I'm perfectly content with them thinking I just have to get closer to some objects to make them out.

So, as I entered middle school I was still that "shy, sheltered, blind kid" who parents love. I remember the first time I heard a peer say a cuss word. I gasped so loudly and long I must have taken in half the oxygen in that room. I put my hand over my mouth and pointed at him (did I mention my private school was also a church?) I immediately ran for the teacher and told on him . . . bad move. Turns out, he was mentally challenged, so the teacher rolled his eyes at me and said sit back down, and the whole class now thought there was something wrong with me. And hence, profanity entered my life.

So did fights, kids smoking, and a whole new knowledge of things I would probably get in trouble for talking about . . . so now, I was just that "shy, blind kid."

Sixth grade, the first year of middle school, was an odd time. I began to realize that my goal of going pro with soccer was unrealistic, so I developed another goal: semi-pro (I was pretty set on this whole soccer thing). It was also a time of simply awful hair—I REFUSED to cut my hair short, and thus I must have tortured the poor barbers with my demands.

Ever since I was 10, I decided I wanted to have that surfer look, so I grew my hair out, but it just didn't turn out to be a surfer look. My hair is thick as can be, and it turned out to be more of a thick, bushy, straight hair afro looking animal that had latched itself to my head. Looking back to the pictures I can't imagine what on Earth I had been thinking. Here is my sixth grade yearbook picture in a nutshell: Afro, barely visible eyes, all while pretty much chewing on my lip and smiling about it. My smile made me look as if I knew something I was not supposed to know—or in great pain, or possibly even on the toilet (no joke). My lower lip was not visible; however, the teeth biting it certainly were. I THOUGHT it would look good. Nope. It was BAD.

Now, here's a little something about my hair. In 5th and 6th grade, it was so long that I literally could not see. And not because of my bad eyes, it was because my hair was covering them. Hence, I was forced to result to hair bands whenever I played soccer, and ONLY when I played soccer. My surfer afro fail was now pushed up by a hidden headband, hidden because I didn't want people to see it. What people *did* see, however, was a large bump at the top of my forehead that followed to wrap around the back, as if there was some sort of weird ring growth, tumor object in the afro animal that had latched itself to my head. On the bright side though, at least I could see to play soccer, right? Well, actually, only sort of.

This is where LHON *really* annoys me, and where this gets a little weird. I do not care about my bad right eye, nor the reduced visual acuity, but what I do care about is a little thing called Ughtoff's disorder. So, with this Ughtoff's disorder, pronounced Yoo-tofs disorder (no need to hack anything up trying to pronounce it), basically both of my eyes suddenly develop massive amounts of small blind spots, and magnify the existing ones due to nerve demyelization. My sight becomes much darker, or dimmer, and it becomes a great deal tougher to see when compared to my normal sight. It all happens very quickly, whenever my body temperature is raised a good amount. So, if I go out with friends in 95 degree weather, I won't be able to see as well. If I play sports in hot weather, I am hopelessly, desperately searching for the dang soccer ball. Even fevers will sometimes trigger this. Until recently, no matter how many times this would happen I could never grow accustomed to it. My family developed the term "dimming" or "going dim" for this occurrence because that is just what happens: the world is literally dimmer. This disorder is not LHON specific though, for it is also common in those with multiple sclerosis.

One way to describe Ughtoff's disorder is by saying it's like fireworks. No single blind spot stays for more than a split second—they flash and vanish very quickly, spanning over the entirety of my vision, which is just plain annoying. One moment my sight is fine enough to see the whole field, next thing I know blind spots are flashing in my eyes and I am desperately searching for the soccer ball. It is quite an odd phenomenon, for the "dimming" can vanish as quickly as it started. One moment my eyes are like fireworks; slap some nice cold water on my face and everything is back to normal (time will also cause it to die down back to normal).

I never really complained or worried about going dim until I began to play soccer at a higher level. I had been playing division 3 and 4 county soccer for about 3 years, and it was just too easy for a few of my teammates. We moved to a different team, and were put on their division 1 team without question. Even division 1 county soccer wasn't hard enough for some of us; a travel team would have been much better, but my family could not accommodate for that sort of lifestyle. Playing at a higher level meant I would have to work harder and perform better—meaning that Ughtoff's was an absolute pain in the butt.

My parents did some research on ways to help me with seeing the soccer ball better, and they found quite possibly the most awesome thing possible for a 12 year old: flipping red-orange sports contacts! (Ohhh, the memories). These contacts would make everything look a shade of orange, but the ball was a vibrant color compared to the background. And, even better, they made my eyes appear bright red to everyone else. I was out on that field with devilish eyes and a new Annapolis Div. 1 jersey on, and as I began to learn the art of being bigger than many of the kids, I started charging around the field, red eyes flashing and pushing people off the ball.

I went on to become the team captain of that team, and every time I went to half-field for the coin flip before each game, I would stare at the other team's captains trying to intimidate them. I probably looked pretty ridiculous, though. I mean, a bright blue and yellow jersey, an exaggerated "tough" face, and eyes that looked as though they were bleeding, all while wearing a hidden head band that make it look as though I had a ring growth on my head probably didn't produce the same effect on the other team as I perceived it would. But, what can I say? It worked for me.

Adding to the list I just mentioned of my absolute fashion disaster, one soccer game I broke my arm. Quite a gory break too—it was pretty nasty. So basically, at the point of my wrist, my hand slid up about 3 inches and my forearm did not line up with my hand. I remember looking down at my arm in awe at how it could do something like that. So now, not only did I have a fabulously terrible look about myself, but I also had a deformed wrist to go along with it.

I did not pull off the "tough" look I was trying to portray into the opponents eyes very well that day. I squealed and screamed and raved over how broken my arm was and cried and sobbed and did every single unmanly thing known to mankind. I was probably sucking my unbroken thumb for all I know. I thought I was gonna die, and I made sure the entire world knew.

Fortunately, I lived and can tell the story of it. Something interesting, though, is that with my eyes, the initial traumatizing moment when I saw my hand was not where it should be and the throbbing and stress kicked in, Ughtoff's kicked in real nicely also. I went dim and the fireworks were everywhere, but when I got off the field, got yelled at a little to calm down, and got some ice, my sight came back just fine (from what I remember . . .). Then my contacts were taken out; apparently we didn't want to freak out the doctors. I really wish my contacts had been left in, though. The doctors would have come in and shouted: "OH MY GOD, GET THIS BOY IN SURGERY!" That would have just made my day.

The red contacts were discontinued, unfortunately, meaning I now had to deal with Ughtoff's disorder without any help from special contacts. This was not all too new to me, for I cannot wear those contacts during gym class (God forbid anyone at school see me in those). In gym class I would just deal with it, and I would NEVER play baseball, as THAT would be a hopeless catastrophe. But I played soccer, basketball, or any other sport with a larger ball just fine. This meant that if I played them in gym just fine, I should be able to perform on the field just fine. That statement held to be true.

I continued soccer just fine without the contacts, but dimming was, and is, still a problem. We went to a doctor about different ways to solve this problem, and we discovered that because this happens when my body is under stress or my body temperature is raised, cooling it would not be a bad idea. We invested in many hand towels and a small cooler. Every practice and game I had, we would fill the cooler with water and ice and put a few hand towels in the cooler. During water breaks I would slap a few of those on my neck and face, then within seconds my sight would be back to the way I normally see. So, there was the solution: ice. However, this does not solve the problem when I have been on the field for a while, but only while I am sitting on the bench. Hence, in my 7th and 8th grade years, a few fruitless attempts were made.

Our theory was that if we could attach multiple ice packs to my body I would remain cold and therefore either minimize the effects of Ughtoff's, or completely eliminate them. So, we set off. A few large, flexible ice packs were bought along with a back brace and a tight T-shirt. We basically wrapped the ice packs around my body and strapped them on me with the back brace—ridiculous. Think of wrapping yourself in freezing ice packs, then putting on a back brace, then a tight t-shirt, and boom. You're "ready" to go play some soccer. It was the most random assortment of items, and they didn't work. If you are curious enough here is what you do: strap the ice packs on as mentioned. Run about ten feet. Turn around. Pick up fallen ice packs from ground. It wasn't the best design.

That method was terrible, and I even used it during one lucky scrimmage (lucky for the parents). Fortunately for me, I had cut my hair a little (a LITTLE. It was still in my eyes a bit), so now I no longer needed my ring growth headband. This is fortunate because that ice pack made my lower

71

back simply bulge. It looked as though I had a birth defect in which my butt grew halfway up my back.

About ten minutes into the scrimmage, I got tired of having to deal with it and just ripped it out, probably earning me many stares from the parents. I mean, one moment you see a kid with a butt halfway up his back, next he is reaching under his shirt, seemingly to scratch this mysterious butt, and out emerges many cloths and a few large white pads (the ice packs). Who wouldn't stare? I wish I was fortunate enough to be a parent on the sidelines, watching a show not performed anywhere else on earth. Attempt #1: Fail.

Attempt two was a little more sensible. We were able to find "ice vests" online, which were made specifically for keeping cool while running in hot weather. The only problem was that I was too embarrassed to wear it. It was a perfect deal—didn't fall off, didn't bounce around much, and did the job. Unfortunately, though, it was big and it was heavy. Running was slower—definitely not good—and hiding it under a jersey was 100 percent out of the question. This vest was popular among my friends who wanted to wear it just for the heck of it, but was not popular with me, the visually-impaired kid who *actually* needed it. Attempt #2: also fail.

Our attempts to keep my vision at my normal while playing sports were unrealistic, and I learned that I would have to just deal with it. By this time, though, in late 7th grade, I no longer wanted to play soccer at any level of a professional. I wanted to go to college and study to become something different, so keeping my vision while playing was no longer as important to me. My academics were now much more important to me, and my goal now was to get into a top college.

I was already in the top classes offered at my school for all 3 years of middle school, with the exception of 7th grade. For some reason, the counselors had placed me in standard science rather than advanced because they were worried about how well I could see chemicals, but this was not a problem because no chemicals were used. The real problem was, and has always been, English. I for one not only suck at English, but also read at a speed normal of those a few years younger than me as result of my eyes. Unfortunately, in English we read from left to right. And unfortunately for me, I have a blind spot directly to the right of my center point of vision in my right eye—meaning that if I were to stare at a single word, the next word would not be visible at all. Hence, I cannot skim very well or read very fast.

In 8th grade they decided that my eyes were not going to be a major problem in science and put me back into advanced science, and my goal was to get straight A's, and to get into a special academic program at my high school. I had decided that I wanted to go to some Ivy League school like Harvard or Princeton, with outrageous prices that I would most likely be paying off for the rest of my life. Yet, two main goals were developed in my last year of middle school: one was to get into the STEM (Science, Technology, Engineering, and Math) program at South River High and two was to make the high school soccer team. I was entering High school feeling confident—I had been accepted into to the STEM program and made the JV soccer team, as a starting striker. The coaches loved me and I loved them. It seemed like nothing could get any better. Ughtoff's disease was also starting to become second nature to me, as it never had before. It was looking to be a bright high school career for me.

Over that summer, the summer of 2010, a catastrophe occurred. My little brother, Grant, informed my family that it was getting hard for him to see. Grant, born only 5 months prior to me losing my sight, was 8 years old when he told my family. My mother scheduled a doctor's appointment, hoping that he just needed glasses. But lo and behold, after the tests were through, there it was: LHON.

August was when LHON became clearly visible in his eyes. His right eye was almost completely blind, and his left eye was quickly following the same path, and for me, school started in late August. He was visiting many doctors and my parents were trying everything to recover his lost sight. It was already predicted for him to slightly recover, as is with some LHON patients, but no guarantee is ensured with this.

As my brother's sight continued to be a major downfall, I stayed focused on a good start to my high school career. As an incoming freshman I had a newfound sense of confidence. It all kicked off busy and quickly—soccer games were twice a week and practices were every day after school, homework started up immediately, and LOTS of it, and a busy schedule with a heavy load was now set upon me. My main focuses became school, soccer, and SLEEP.

For many years, probably ever since I myself had begun to lose my sight, my mother always wanted us to visit LHON specialists. In September of 2010, when the effects of LHON were clearly visible on my brother, she scheduled an appointment my brother and I in California to see these specialists. It was a well worth trip, seeing as my parents wanted ANY options to help with my little bro's eyes.

So, what happened at this doctor's appointment? Well, first there were many eye tests, with my brother especially, many talks with doctors, and in the end, my brother was sent home with a box full of some funky, EXPENSIVE (yet free for us) medicine. Actually, I don't even know what to call this. I don't know if this qualifies as "medicine," because I consider medicine as something for when you're sick with maybe a cold, flu, or even cancer—not for when you are blind, but oh well. Nobody has ever been cured after having actual nerve damage and lost vision, but heck, this stuff was worth a shot. And speaking of things worth a shot, that same September after we flew out to California, I spotted a shot well worth taking. That September I met this blonde haired blue eyed smart girl who I suddenly had a huge crush on. Somehow, talking to her was not a difficult task, and after much pressure from friends, I asked her out and we began to date.

My brother had received some stuff that we hoped may aid his eyes and, well, I did not. But, I now had girl to date, and school and soccer could not be better. Jen and I have been dating for about 2 years now, and I will never forget that eventful September where my little bro was given that little piece of hope. As freshman year progressed, things just got better.

That winter, I went out for the indoor track team. In soccer I was always the quickest runner and whenever I got the ball, I would pretty much run straight down the field trucking over people as I went. So, for track I wanted to be a sprinter. Sprinting did not turn out to be my forte, and neither was distance running. I settled into the "middle distance" section, which were events that were short and quick, but not all out sprints. The 400m dash and 800m run turned out to be my main events.

As the season progressed, my performance improved until soon I was competing with the upper classmen for spots on relays and in events, and the next thing I knew, I was running varsity track as a freshman on the 4x400m relay team (4 people each run 400 meters). I was dumbfounded, and had quite an exciting season with them.

Making varsity track was awesome, but it just kept getting better as the year progressed. As a part of STEM, we are required to enter contests, and our advisor, Mrs. Lesko, informed us of a contest that we were required to participate in. The contest was called the "Invent an Instrument" contest, sponsored by the Blue Man group (a bunch of dudes who cover themselves in blue paint and put on a pretty wicked show), and it was a contest throughout the USA. In addition to entering the national contest, we were to have our own little contest within just STEM.

Basically, the contest was to design and make an instrument out of everyday items, such as spoons, bottles, rubber bands—basically anything. Then, videotape yourself with the instrument showing how it worked, and submit it on the Blue Man website. The grand prize was $5,000 for the winner, $5,000 for their school, four tickets to Orlando, and the chance to see your instrument played onstage during a live concert. When our advisor told my class about the contest, she threw in that she truly believed that someone in our program would win the competition. We pretty much sat there and laughed, not believing it to be possible.

I got started the very day we were told about the contest. I designed on paper what I wanted to create, and modified it as I found things around the house. Long story short, my final design included a five gallon paint bucket, rubber bands stretched across the top of the bucket that could be plucked to make a pitch, and a method of hitting the base of the bucket to produce a deep, drum-like beat.

I decided that I was going to mount the bucket on a platform using wooden dowels (basically wood rods) so that the entire bucket was raised about a foot in the air. From there, I would attach a foot pedal that when pressed would cause a padded dowel to rise up and hit the base of the bucket. I discovered that this design had an extra benefit—as a result of the bucket being mounted and raised, I could play the strings with two hands. I had the ability to pinch the rubber bands with one hand to shorten or lengthen the length of the bands, therefore creating a wide variety of pitches that could be produced.

I felt like a flipping genius after I had it all drawn out on paper with a plan to build it, and the construction of it was a chore, but it got done. I called it "the Base Guitar Drum" . . . so creative, right? Well, I didn't really care much about winning the national contest as it wasn't really realistic to me. Someone else would certainly design something better, (right?), but the STEM competition, well maybe. After all, my invention was pretty darn "cool".

I submitted my video of myself showing off my contraption, and playing the song "Seven Nation Army" by the White Stripes—the perfect song for this instrument.

One morning at school, I got called down to the STEM main room in the school. I thought I was about to get grilled about something or was in some sort of trouble, but as I walked into the room, I was greeted by a loud applause from many of my classmates—DEFINITELY trouble. As I look around the room, I see my family standing at the front with my ridiculous instrument, and looking to my right, there is my girlfriend sitting there with a camera in her hand waving. Then I saw a news channel camera crew next to my family . . . oh God, what was this all about? I thought I maybe won the little contest within only STEM, and thought all this was a BIT overkill.

"You have just won the grand prize for the National Invent an Instrument Contest, Chase Rudisill" . . . .

"WHAT?!" How the #%$& did that happen?? Did I just win five grand? Apparently. Am I going to Orlando?—Yep . . ." . . . cool . . ." Needless to say, it did not hit me until later, and as I got interviewed by a news crew, I am pretty sure I said I would use my money on a "cawer . . . hehe." I could not even think or say the word car, and what's weird is I didn't even want to spend it on a "cawer." I was walking on clouds, though—I probably looked like I was on dentist meds. The bell rang and I flipping sprinted out of that classroom, high fiving random people and hugging my friends, getting shouts across the hallway—it was awesome. It was something I would have never dreamed of when I was younger and I mean, I was 15. It was a bit overwhelming to hear so much.

I went on to run varsity outdoor track, and became a main part of the 4x800m relay (4 people, each run 800 meters) and the 4x400m relay. We again had a mediocre season, but that's OK because at the end of the season I was going to Orlando for 4 days! About a month before I left, though, my winnings of the contest changed a little. The Blue Man Group told me they were unable to figure out how to tune and play my instrument. I was informed that I would not be watching them play my instrument on stage anymore . . . I would be playing it. Now, not only did I have five grand, free tickets to Orlando, and had won a bunch of money for my school, but I would be playing on stage with the Blue Man Group in front of a huge crowd!

I was so incredibly nervous I could not sit still. I knew the song I'd be playing onstage well, so that was alright, but being worried of tripping onstage wasn't helping. The stage was pitch black and full of wires—big ones too. At that point, I had to tell them I was visually impaired to avoid my own personal embarrassment of tripping and face-planting probably, with my luck, right into my bucket instrument. They would need to move a few wires around.

The experience was exhilarating—I did not expect nearly as loud of a roar from the crowd as I received. But a good song with the Blue Man Group and a good cheer from the crowd amounted to one heck of a day. Later, I was given one of those huge checks for five thousand dollars on stage, and that currently is sitting in my room, cherished and loved by myself.

Two varsity letters, all A's and one B, a national contest champion, an award from the Maryland Senate for winning the contest, and an attractive girlfriend, I was feeling pretty successful—and sophomore year was not a bad follow up.

One of my more unique experiences happened in November of my sophomore year. As part of STEM, a group of 2 others and I had to enter a science fair. We decided to attempt to lengthen the amount of time an electrical scooter would run through attaching a car alternator to the battery. We should have done more research though, for we in fact cut the lifetime of the scooter in half, rather that extending it, in the end. It was one of the biggest learning experiences of my life, for we had many faults:

Fault #1: We did not even hook the alternator to the battery. Actually, we hooked it up to the completely wrong spot. Fault #2: The alternator was not even generating electricity. Fault #3: We exceeded the scooter's max weight by about 70 pounds. And lastly, fault #4 was actually a blessing in disguise, if we *had* managed to hook up the alternator correctly, and *had* managed to get the alternator to generate electricity; we would have blown ourselves and the scooter up. We had too many volts leading to lead acid batteries—we were bound to blow something up. Unless you're not a teenage idiot like us, don't mess with batteries. We ended up getting second place in our section for the regional science fair for our, what should have been titled, "blow yourself up" project.

In the winter, I ran indoor track and this season was even better than last year's. Within the first few meets, the coaches had figured out the A teams (equivalent to first string players in other varsity sports) for the relays. I was on the A 4x400m team, and the A 4x800m team. The 4x800m team was where it was at. We were just a mere 3.5 seconds away from the indoor track school record, and were almost sent to states. Unfortunately, one of us became sick so we had to run our alternate in the qualifying regional meet and could not quite make the time, but that only intensified our want for states in the outdoor track season that spring.

That winter I made my second trip out to California, tagging along with my brother because he went out there about every 3 months. We went out with high hopes to get me on the same medicine my brother had received. But there was no longer an option to receive the medicine. The only option was to join a trial that was to be conducted. My chances of getting the real stuff over the placebo were 50 percent. Unfortunately, the trial was cancelled due to multiple factors.

We had one other option when we got the news that I could not have the medicine, and that was to go to Brazil to try for it. (Ummm, yes please!). Apparently Brazil was currently still issuing the medicine, and we were trying to get me into the studies in Brazil. Unfortunately, after further phone calls and research, we discovered I could not get it in Brazil either.

It was a disappointing winter, having lost the opportunity to go to states with my 4x800m team by mere seconds, and I did not return from California with some funky meds. But oh well, spring was rolling around and outdoor track started quickly, with better results than the indoor season.

My 4x800m team was increasingly getting better as we went, and long story short, we placed second in the region qualifying for states. Running in the state championship meet was an amazing experience, and my relay came in 11th place in the state of Maryland. Even better was that we were a very young team and have another full year together, and just as the track season had taken a turn for the better, so had my academics.

I have had a good life plus first two years of high school, and I cannot complain about my visual impairment much. I was cleared for my learner's permit, and will have my driver's license this upcoming November of 2012. The doctor informed us there were people with much worse vision from Glaucoma, cataracts, etc, who also qualify legally to drive. How does it feel knowing a visually challenged guy is going to be driving? Safe, huh? Think about that the next time you venture out the door!

I have had good grades, two great soccer seasons, have 4 varsity letters, have 6 medals and 7 ribbons from track, plus one participation in a state championship, won a national contest, have $5,000, have an award from the Maryland Senate, placed second in a regional science fair, and LHON is just another part of me.

Where am I today? Well, I am currently the "control" variable in a medical paper being published on my brother as he takes the funky meds he got in California that I myself was NOT able to get. Let me tell you, knowing I will be a subject for a major medical paper to be published is nice and all, but how am I being mentioned? As the freaking CONTROL! And just for reference, the control is an identical group to the treatment group that does not receive any of the treatment being tested in order to compare what the effects of the treatment are to what would normally happen (my brother and I are considered identical twins in mitochondrial DNA because we have the same mother). I would much rather be in the "treatment" group, not the "control" group. In this case, I sit and take the same tests my brother does to show that any change in his eyes are works of the medicine, not just mere coincidence. All I can say right now is I *hope* whatever they write is convincing, because I want that medicine to be released for the use of others *soon*.

Chase Rudisill

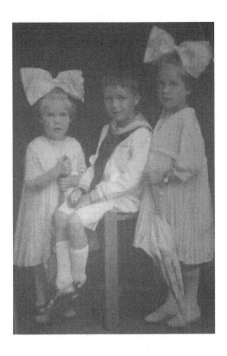

The Curious Man with the
Odd Magnifying Glass

There goes the curious man walking down the street again. The neighbors are peering out through their curtains and wondering, "What is he doing?" It was an experiment. It was the early 1950's and the new televisions were the rage. Only problem, the large screens were actually 7 inches. No one can see a 7 inch screen, much less George who had vision loss. Jack Benny, Red Skelton, and Uncle Miltie are all easier to see from behind the 12 inch magnifying glass which George had. The glass is thick, maybe 5 to 6 inches thick. One side magnifies and the other side reduces the image. George was experimenting. Did the glass help him see more? Which side worked to expand his field of vision: the concave or the convex?

George was the first born child of Doc Stephan and his young wife, Rose. He was such a handsome child, beautiful in every way imaginable. The year was 1912. He had the good fortune of arriving into a wealthy family. Two sisters came into the family 2 years and 4 years later, followed by a brother. The family was a military family serving at Fort Hancock in Georgia during World War I. They lived on a farm. The children had a beloved nanny. Their life was idyllic.

After the War they returned to their home in Atglen, PA. They lived an affluent life as Doc Stephan was the only doctor in town. At first he went on house calls, day and night, sunshine and rain, by horse and buggy. When the gasoline powered automobiles were introduced, they had the first one in town. They also had the first telephone.

The Great Depression came, but the family was still able to send George, Jr., to fine Universities, to study medicine and follow in his father's footsteps. George would be a successful and prosperous physician. He attended Bucknell University, University of Alabama, and Duke University. He never finished. Near the end of his schooling, George was losing his sight. George was only 26 years old. He drove to his sister, Elizabeth's, home in Germantown, PA. He sat on the edge of the bed with his head in his hands as he explained to her and her husband, Baird, what was happening.

His father, Doc Stephan, who was now head of Jefferson Medical Hospital in Philadelphia, was contacted. His father had him admitted to the hospital and many tests were performed. There were three months of studies. Occasionally LHON presents with symptoms similar to Multiple Sclerosis (MS). Wills Eye doctors studied his eyes. It was announced George had MS. By this time, a controlling and adversarial stepmother, Ruth, had replaced the children's natural mother. Ruth pronounced George (probably) was drinking bathtub gin while at the University of Alabama. This, according to her, caused George's loss of sight. The first sad event for George was the early death of his mother from pneumonia; the second event was now his loss of sight, followed then by a step-mother spreading horrible rumors.

LHON had first been discovered in 1883 by Dr. Leber. Since Will's Eye was the top eye hospital in the world, it is hard to believe George was not diagnosed with LHON. There are two issues that surround the misdiagnosis: one medical and one familial. As far as the medical diagnosis theory, everyone before 1883 was misdiagnosed. Even after that, hundreds if not thousands of patients across the globe continued to receive inaccurate assessments of the cause of their blindness. There are patients still suffering today who have absolutely no clue why they are blind. Follow-up visits become futile, so access to new information can be limited. Considering the United States' status of being highly developed, most patients and eye doctors have gained a considerable greater amount of exposure to LHON than those located in Third World countries, so misdiagnosis is less common. It is amazing that George and so many others have lived their lives suffering from a disease of which they only knew the effects and not the cause.

The second hypothesis is purely familial. Is it possible that the top eye hospital correctly diagnosed George and his father chose to hide the information from the family? The purpose of this would have been for the perceived benefit of George's siblings. George's father had two daughters and another son. Who would want to marry them? Who would want to have children with them? A future wife might not be interested in a blind husband and likewise would a future husband want blind children, or a blind wife and blind children? No one is around to confirm or deny this so one can only speculate. But potentially, mothers and fathers would be "stuck" with spinster daughters who carried these genes.

George met and married the young widow Ethel who had a 6 year old daughter. His father helped them buy a small farm in Lancaster County to support their growing family. First a son, George III, was born. Baby George had Down's syndrome. What more did George, Jr. need on his plate? Two more sons, perfectly healthy, were born in close succession. Then Ethel was pregnant again. The children were demanding. Once, George III swallowed a nipple because it wasn't secure on the bottle. While they had farm hands to help with the chores, it was more than the young couple could handle. One evening, the distraught and exhausted nine month pregnant Ethel took a stroll along the creek on the farm. Ethel never returned. The family helped search for days and eventually her lifeless body was found in the creek. The children went to live with their maternal grandmother. The farm went to foreclosure.

George went for training with the School for the Blind. He learned to make straw brooms. Then he was sent out on the streets to sell brooms and pencils. This was a long way from being the prominent medical student he once was.

George went to live with his sister Elizabeth, her husband Baird, and their two children Leslie and Larry. George drove the children to distraction by sitting between them and the magnifying glass used for the TV. Always though, George remained the children's favorite relative, because he had a wonderful sense of humor and they were in constant laughter.

Elizabeth and Baird lost their home to Sheriff Sale and had to move to rented homes. They were all homeless and George had to go to stay with whomever would give him a place to lay his head. They all stayed close to each other. Baird and George were particularly good friends. Elizabeth and Baird never believed the bathtub gin stories about George. However, in later years George did become an alcoholic in his 40's. He died of heart failure in his early 50's, never knowing what he truly had, LHON 14484. George was penniless and the family had to pitch in for his burial.

Elizabeth also did not know George had LHON, until her grandson began to lose his sight. She denied for years that it could have been a gene from her. She said her "mother would be sick" to know George's plight. Her father had the finest doctors study his condition. At one point Elizabeth wanted to have George exhumed, to prove he didn't have a defective gene. Sometimes family members feel guilty about passing down a hereditary condition. Eventually, after more than 5 years, she came to accept the information. She had inherited the gene from her mother, passed it to her daughter, who has now passed it to her granddaughter and grandsons, and her great-granddaughter and great-grandsons currently carry her gene.

GEORGE LOUIS STEPHAN, JR.
Presented by his niece: Leslie Stone Byrne
PENNSYLVANIA 1912-1964

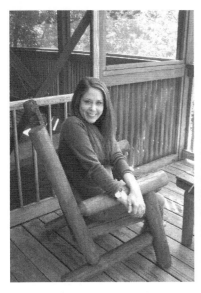

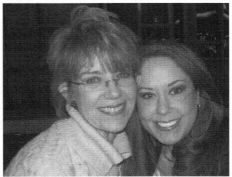

Legally Blind

It was the beginning of a beautiful spring in Southeast Texas. I had been summoned to design and dig a garden at a friend's bay-front property. This was helped by the fact that I bragged about having been so good at similar projects back home. I loved digging in the dirt and clearly remember the intensity of the colors of those flowers and plants I put in the earth. Although it was about to change, life at that moment with spring anew was exhilarating and beautiful around me. I had on everything I needed for that week or so: gardening gloves, flip-flops, shorts, a bikini top and, of course, sunglasses. The sun glared so brightly off that water; the bulkhead of the bay was only fifteen feet away.

Over several days, I began experiencing what I thought was a reaction to having the full sun in my eyes. I couldn't explain it. On about the third day of this, I remember calling my mom and relating to her that I was trying to look at the lines between a set of mini-blinds but when I looked directly at the blinds I saw what looked like one big pull-down shade. Any detail faded and I could not focus.

Very soon after, I drove what was to be my last long distance trip. I went from this waterfront house in tiny Oak Island, Texas, to meet my mom and future stepfather, Tom, in Austin, Texas, on their trip from my home state of Tennessee. This was on March 23, 2008, Easter Sunday, two weeks before my 28th birthday. The trip was planned before the sudden blurriness, so I struggled to see the road both coming and going as I drove. I somehow remember knowing this would be my final journey of independence for a long while.

One of my last and best-sighted memories while on that vacation is at the state museum in Austin with my Mom, watching a holographic visually intense presentation about the history of the State of Texas. I wonder if it seems so magical and intense only now because it was one of my last sighted memories. Our next day at the Alamo was enjoyable, but I couldn't make out the curator's face during his oral retelling of its history.

My mom and I seemed to cling to each other that trip as if we knew how much strength we would need to draw from each other in the near future. I left Mom and Tom early, so as to use every bit of daylight to drive back toward Houston—my sight was fading so quickly. In the ensuing weeks, my mother checked with me every day to see if my sight was improving. With increasing confusion and dread I continued to tell her it was not.

In just a week's span of time from returning from that trip I was at my first appointment at Houston Eye Associates. The facility was huge and came highly recommended and I felt positive I would find an answer. What I found was frustration. It ran both ways. Every time a technician would put lenses in front of my eyes, switch them and ask if one was better than the other, I responded "no." They acted as though I wasn't concentrating or trying. They didn't understand there was no way any corrective lens could help this blurriness.

I explained that my vision was as though an object I looked at completely faded away into the background. Everything was very indiscernible. It looked as though I had just looked into bright oncoming headlights and then looked away: not a full image in my central vision as one gets when one looks at the sun and looks away, but a constant terrible glare you cannot look away from.

Initially, when I explained this condition first happened after exposure to direct sunlight, the doctor suggested I purchase dark, polarized sunglasses and cover all windows in hopes that this would quickly ease possible photokeratitis. This is commonly known as "welder's flash" or "snow blindness." Unlike in these cases my vision wasn't returning.

Additionally, x-rays revealed a hairline fracture on my brow bone from a fall I had in my kitchen months earlier. I slipped and hit my head on my dog's porcelain bowl that resulted in a black eye. My doctor thought, perhaps, that I had a pinched nerve or maybe pressure behind the eye or a myriad of other problems that steroids might help. I took rounds of Prednisone. By this time I was having to write in giant print and was posting a schedule of days and milligrams associated with the steroids on my refrigerator. I called my mom every day and stood a specific number of feet away from my microwave's clock readout hoping to be able to step inches back and still see the time. Instead I had to inch closer to figure it out.

My mom started taking time from her teaching job and flew to Houston frequently to go to ophthalmologists and doctor appointments with me. Our delight in seeing each other was marred by worry. We made the best of day-long appointments with humor and anything to divert our thoughts from what was happening to me. Tests were negative for both multiple sclerosis and diabetes—both being possible explanations for the sudden sight loss. MRI and CAT scans showed nothing.

I began drinking heavily at this time. I had no idea what was happening. I was scared to death. I didn't want to live my days in this confusing new blurry world. I wanted to feel blurry on the inside. I didn't want my emotions to be sharp. My mom and those around me did not know this. The constant worry and confusion just made me sound upset all the time. My mom, and others, all stayed positive about a resolution. We thought medicine had answers for everything. And we thought answers meant cures. My mom even sent me some "Get Well Soon" cards that students in her class made for me during this trying time—in giant print, of course.

In exhaustive frustration, after about five months of fruitless tests, the doctor at Houston Eye Associates suggested to my mother that it was "all in my head." It was then that my mom found a neuro-ophthalmologist (the seventeenth and final doctor in my search for an answer) at Baylor College of Medicine in Houston, Texas. On September 17, 2008, all confidence and hope for a cure was smashed when I learned of LHON strain number 11778 through the DNA test results.

My best and longtime family friend, Colin, with whom I was living in Houston, took me to this final appointment, as well as this search from optometrists to ophthalmologists to neurologist to neuro-ophthalmologist and the whole gamut of labs in between. The doctor told me very coldly and concisely that I had "Leber's" and that Colin and I should, "Write that down and write the strain number, too." In his next sentence he stated that there was no cure, and it was very rare, that it was mostly in males, and that it was passed maternally. His next sentence was that I too would pass this to any future children.

How did I spend the remainder of that day? I drank and cried. My mom was sitting in a school faculty meeting in Tennessee—a thousand miles from me—waiting for my phone call. I'll never forget calling her and uttering the words "It's genetic" and saying my brother's name as well to her (the gene was passed to him, too) and hearing my mother wail a resounding, "NO!" I later learned in her tireless research regarding my symptoms that Mom had read about the possibility of LHON. We were all crushed by this diagnosis. We had waited so long for an answer, only to feel that "Team Hope" had lost in overtime.

With nowhere to turn for information, we were on our own to fend for answers over the Internet. We found my symptoms and age of onset were much like other cases of LHON—except for my being female. My mom immediately found an on-line support group where even if answers weren't to be had, at least others were converging and sharing their experiences. I had no idea how those people were even communicating on-line. I looked at my computer and cried. It was an obsolete reminder of my newly acquired disability. I felt jealous that my mom had found support through the very thing I was no longer capable of using. This especially bothered me in its cruel irony. I felt like *I* was the one—the affected one—who needed support. I resented the fact she got to lean on other carriers. This was the first tinge of anger at my mom that later manifested in a particularly terrible outburst of rage on my 29th birthday, while she was visiting me in Houston (which I will later discuss).

In retrospect, I don't know how I would have made it through this period without the support of loved ones and professionals committed to helping people like me. I was slowly taken from point A to point B in approaching how to live as a new legally-blind person. As I sat in self-pity and deep depression, drinking through the day, those who loved me were helping me put one foot in front of the other. They seemed to realize that life goes on, whereas I believed it to be over. I now know this was God doing for me what I could not do for myself.

My mom was my biggest cheerleader. She told me that although my character was being put to the test, she was sure I could make it to the other side of this madness. She could only sympathize with what I was going through, but understood that it was devastatingly painful. I don't think anyone expected me to be immediately functional as a severally visually-impaired person. This is why Mom would say things like, "It WILL get better." Or reference the FUTURE. The Texas Department of Assistive and Rehabilitative Services (DARS) opened a case for me. An outline of services and therapy was made. Completion of my case gave this "FUTURE" of semi-normality an estimated date.

I drifted, defeated and drunk, through basic introduction of assisted technology and devices. Every week I wailed, heartbroken, to a state-provided therapist who assumed I had Post-Traumatic Stress Disorder. I remember crumpling in the driveway on the day my car finally sold as the taillights faded off, knowing that part of my independence was leaving forever, too. It was Christmas 2008—just three months after getting the diagnosis that revealed to me that I would no longer be doing something I still miss most to this day—driving. Now living in a house with Colin (initially I'd only gone to Texas to enjoy a few months' stay!), he was increasingly gone out of town for work without even a car in the driveway to represent someone being home. I disappeared so much in that house emotionally that there really wasn't anyone at home. If being a person requires having a soul, that house was vacant. I became completely dead inside. The selling of my car represented such a final tragedy for me. It wasn't that I could just no longer read my mail, use the computer, see my face in the mirror, or even watch television! Now I had lost the ability to decide when and where I would go, too! At 28, I had backtracked in independence to my early teens. My increased alcoholism took an especially bad turn for the worse from that moment on.

No matter how defeated I felt, though, I didn't let the lack of a car keep me from getting to the liquor store. I was monumentally struggling with being a full-blown alcoholic and, at the same time, attempting to complete my case with DARS. I simply refused to accept that this was now my fate: Learn how to balance a checkbook blind? Figure out personal hygiene for the severely visually impaired? This was someone else's life! And you've got to be kidding about using that white cane! Nevertheless, I attempted classes at the DARS building in downtown Houston. But I found my body was so terribly addicted to alcohol, by this time, I had to drink shots in the morning to stop the shakes and keep from being sick for the day. Everywhere I went I had a Gatorade bottle in my purse that was half-filled with vodka. This amount meant that I couldn't be gone from my home very long to any kind of casework, class, or therapist without the shakes starting. I only went to these appointments and straight back home. I had no friends, so I never went to bars to sit alone. Someone would figure out I was blind and then wouldn't want to be with me. Also, I couldn't bear the humiliation of having someone read a restaurant menu to me like they would to a child. I couldn't manage the grocery store (not wanting to ask for help) and I ate very little. It was difficult to explain to a clerk that my normal looking blue eyes couldn't see anything in the store. All the confusion and frustration shown to me by employees everywhere I went only increased my desire to resign further from the outside world. I was never fall-down drunk outside of the house, just intoxicated enough to make this terrible reality seem like it was just a dream. Every day, when I woke up and opened my eyes, and realized that the real world was out of sight, unlike the full-vision dream I had just had, I just wanted to fade back out again. Being a Christian, I couldn't even find solace in church, as I couldn't make it through a service without a drink to get me through.

I was at one particular class at the DARS building when I found I could no longer separate my alcoholic thought process from class participation. This class was about job interview skills for the blind. Of course, in retrospect, I probably misunderstood the speakers. In my muddled mind, I heard them say to be overly gracious for even having the opportunity to be interviewed. It was so obvious to me that the choice of job I wanted in life was now gone. I had excelled in college to find myself, only six years later, being told to *hope* for a kind soul willing to take me on, ride the bus with my cane to get there and beg for what I saw as *philanthropy*. My alcoholism was screaming in my head, "Get out of here! You can't do this. Go home and disappear. You can't see people, why should they see you?" Several hours into class, smiling on the outside, scoffing on the inside, and with the beginning of my daily Delirium Tremens (DTs), I approached the front of the room with my cane (my prop that said, "I'm participating") and made up something about a toothache and left. Soon after, my DARS counselor came to my house and said I smelled of alcohol at the class and that it wasn't the first time. I was asked to scrawl my signature on one of their forms saying I was on thirty-day's probation to stop drinking or services would be cancelled. I signed it, still knowing I couldn't stop. I didn't admit defeat and ask my counselor for help, like I could have. I just wanted her and the whole idea of living like this gone. This was early spring 2009—the one year anniversary since the loss of my sight—and the rest of me was dying inside, too.

Colin knew I was heavily drinking to mask the pain. Mom suspected, but never to the degree that I did (toward the end, a fifth of vodka per day). They both tell me they don't stand in judgment of me because no one knows how they will react until faced with similar tribulation. My alcoholism was severe, but no one had the heart to tell me to take on this issue, when the more pressing matter at hand was that of living blind. No one knew that alcohol would soon surpass LHON as the most devastating thing in my life.

My mom came to Houston for my 29th birthday, on 7 April 2009. Until that day, I had never outright blamed or been angry with her for supplying the maternally-passed defective gene. I'd asked God "why" in teary outbursts many times, yet never felt anger at Him. On that particular day, though, my rage was finally let loose.

She and Colin took me to dinner and as I sat and listened to them chat about a world of which I was no longer a part, the hate inside me swelled to the surface. How dare my mom be happy and not sad forever like me! I couldn't share in their genuine laughter because there was none left to be had in my heart. When we got home I unleashed a fury of verbal abuse to my mother. Everything she had ever done in my life to upset me I was now angry about all over again. How could she have wasted even a minute of my sighted life being imperfect? I felt an old feeling I had suppressed all over again. I felt that I was always the child, between my brother and me, who had taken the most punishment growing up and now she was doing it all over again.

91

I felt I had been very screwed in the deal of being her daughter. I blamed her for giving me this horrible disease that took my sight and robbed me of the best years of my life to come. In my mind my life was over and she had ruined it.

I behaved so poorly that even in a drunken haze I still remembered my mom's heartbroken cries. I kicked her out of my house and out of my life. We were truly in the middle of the tempest that would test our relationship's strength. This is a terrible memory and with so many other memories gone, I suppose I kept this one so I can share its message of hope in these pages. She has forgiven me, finding comfort in knowing that anger is a crucial stage of the grieving process. I know my alcoholism flared this already volatile fire. I understand she is not alone in having been blamed for a child's LHON. I can only hope those relationships have healed as immensely as ours has.

Although Mom and I barely spoke after that, she was instrumental in finding and getting me in the clinical LHON study at Bascom Palmer Eye Institute at the University of Miami, School of Medicine, for my first appointment in June of that year. As it happened, the doctor at Houston Eye Associates who had incorrectly diagnosed my LHON felt compelled to find a direction in which to point us in. At home all day now, I was there to receive an unexpected call from him and he asked to get my mother on the line in Tennessee. I did so and he told her of a doctor who was conducting studies on gene therapy. He'd heard of her work at a seminar he attended and was reminded of me. A call to Dr. Jean Bennett in Pennsylvania ultimately led us to call Dr. John Guy at the University of Miami. She explained my situation and he immediately wanted me in the study.

My longtime, on-again, off-again, boyfriend, Jeff, met me in Miami in June to accompany me for the overnight stay and all-day testing appointment. He was aware of my destitute situation and we made sure my trusty Gatorade bottle was never far. My need for drink exceeded the supply I took to the eye institute that day and I was soon in agony; vomiting on the bathroom floor, having sent Jeff with cab fare and liquor money out the door with pleading cries for him to hurry. I only held on to finish the appointment because I was already there, and knew that if they kicked me out of the study my hope for sight restoration treatment would be gone.

That one June appointment at Bascom Palmer was the only thing of importance in my life and once it was over, my thoughts of Mom's last visit haunted me once more. I never recovered emotionally from "losing it" with her, and decided to completely stop trying. Every moment that I wasn't already in drunken oblivion, I was drinking to get there. I didn't leave my house again except to go to the liquor store and soon was incapable of doing that. On the rare occasion that Colin was home to drive me to the store, I would buy enough vodka to last me for weeks. He started going to the liquor store for me and never said no when I asked, because he knew I would somehow get there. By June, I was in no shape to even get up from the bed. I only slept in passed-out spurts and those were only for a few hours at a time before the nausea and panic of the DTs would wake me. If my talking watch said it was four o'clock, I had no idea if that meant AM or PM. Concerned neighbors would ring my doorbell not knowing I was on the other side—too sick to move. Most of my bodily functions took place in and around my bed with its night table as a stocked bar.

In addition to seeing a therapist, I had been under the care of a general practitioner. I had blood work done and he told me I was severely alcoholic with very unsafe liver enzyme levels and increasing alcohol—induced peripheral neuropathy in my legs and feet (the neuropathy is apparently irreversible damage because the constant pang is still daily for me). He told me to stop drinking, but since my case with DARS didn't depend on his input, I was honest and told him that wasn't an option for me. It was asking me to do something I truly believed wasn't ever going to happen. The daily pain for the few hours a day my body sobered up through sleep or some "handicapped" training was too great to fathom sticking it out for any length of time.

I fell every time I walked and was bruised all over my body. I had been bruising from falls at home since the heavy drinking had begun, but I looked especially bad now. The bruising was amplified by diagnosed anemia from poor nutrition. During this time I rarely ate, ingesting little but alcohol. My body screamed for me to feed it. My pleading stomach sometimes convinced me to go stumbling, and even crawling, to the refrigerator. I gorged but I was emaciated because I drank to the point of frequent vomiting.

I vaguely remember this, but the power went out in a storm on a summer night during one of Colin's absences. My mind must have been gone from sheer alcohol poisoning at this time, but, for the life of me, I could not find my way around my house. I crawled and used the bathroom and passed out wherever for that whole night. The king size box springs and mattress, on the floor of that giant master bedroom, is where my body barely functioned enough to drink and survive for those couple of months. I vomited in the trashcan beside me. If it was full or knocked over, it just went on the floor. As my color blindness prohibits me from seeing red, I could not even see that I was constantly vomiting blood. Soon I found myself unable to walk, as my leg muscles had atrophied. I wheeled myself about the house on an office chair. The couple of weeks just before July 15th I didn't leave the bed for anything at all—not *anything*.

My ugly home phone with its giant buttons and long tangled cord was always on the bed with me and rang constantly, though I often ignored it or unplugged it from the wall. I knew I wouldn't live long like this but didn't care—never concerned that my death would hurt others. I couldn't have gotten better for them anyway—I was too far gone. I never thought I could recover from what happened to me: developing this damned LHON, or the now fatal alcoholism that ensued. I was lying there in that spot, life now hell on earth and in-between blackouts, at two AM on 15 July 2009, when the phone rang. Answering it became the first step in what I can only explain as divine intervention. It was my mom. Even totally drunk, I managed to be a smart-ass to her. I still hated her for "giving me" LHON. She had asked me not to call her past 10 PM (something I was noted for with repeated "suicide" calls) and at that hour I asked her why she was breaking her own rule (the alcoholic mind—demanding respect and equality while drinking oneself to the grave). She said she was worried about me and asked if I was okay. Only God sending the voice of my heartbroken mother could make me crumple like a weeping child and confess—if just for an instant—an actual fear of dying. I answered and said: "No, mommy, I'm not. I'm sick." She asked my permission to call DARS as soon as they opened and send someone out to check on me. I don't remember anything after this, but I know that 911 summoned an ambulance to my house.

Then: a big blank. My last few memories (until much later in August) are of lying in the emergency room and being with Deb, my mobility (white cane) therapy counselor (whom my mother summoned that morning), who helped me so much that year. I was awake and talking to the paramedics. They could see I was malnourished and intoxicated. They were astonished at my body's frailty and appearance. They were shocked at my severe bruises. They were dumbfounded with my ambiguous answers. In my insanity, I honestly thought if I acted right I would get some necessary fluids and go home soon where I would drink—but definitely less. I even called Colin and asked him to bring me a "special" water bottle (meaning one consisting of straight vodka). I was well aware of the terror of too much alcohol leaving my system. He ignored my plea and just said he was on his way.

As tests started coming back revealing my condition as critical, and as time slowly passed, my temperature plummeted. I remember not being allowed to cover up with blankets and I was shaking violently. I had been denying long-term abuse, and of course its severity, since I got there. My heart was racing. There was no denying that this was anything but very bad. The physicians were telling Deb about admitting me immediately and calling my mother. I insisted they not. I was awake but completely freaking out when I heard the physicians preparing to put tubes, of some type, down my throat through my nose. I know now they were leaving my throat clear for surgery to repair a bad tear in my esophagus.

Deb was allowed to stay at the foot of my bed rubbing my feet. She explained who she was to help shed light on how I got there. I was having a full-blown panic attack and deadly DTs. She asked me what my favorite place in the world was. She asked me what my favorite food was. And as I experienced the most painful thing to this day in my life—the insertion of that ventilator down my nose—she told my answers right back to me in a beautiful story. She described me sitting on the back porch of my Mama's (my maternal grandmother), looking out at the barn and eating her fried chicken. In the background there was some nervous talk about my heart rate. The next thing I heard was the sound of my mother's voice. The same voice from those early morning hours—but it was weeks later. After learning what happened, I know that I can tell you my first real memory of her being there with me, talking to me is after I was awakened from a second induced coma. I remember nothing before that, but felt like I had been expecting her to be there, when she woke me up whispering, so many days later.

[The following account is by my mother, Sandra Kanon]:

"Moon River, wider than a mile . . ." Over and over I sang those poignant Johnny Mercer lyrics to her as I stroked Catherine's vomit-matted hair, remembering how I'd rocked her to sleep as a baby, singing of Moon River and dreaming of a much different rainbow's end than the one I now feared was eminent. I kissed her swollen, bloated cheek and wondered where in this almost unrecognizable form my strikingly beautiful daughter had retreated. I lifted her left hand and kissed the scar on her pinky finger, remembering the bike wreck that gave her a boxer's fracture at age 12 and wished so badly that now at 29 she could fight her way out of this darkness of despair and survive. Sitting here with her now—watching her in a coma—I began to recount the desperate details that brought me to this moment . . . .

It was 8 PM on the night of July 15, 2009. I was at Tom's apartment. My cell phone rang and I saw that it was Catherine's number. Quickly answering, I was somewhat taken aback when the voice on the other end was a man's: "This is Dr. Maher calling from the ER at Christus St. Catherine Hospital." I remember sinking to the floor when he told me Catherine was in very bad condition and was being given a 50/50 chance of surviving the night. He mentioned a torn esophagus . . . severe malnutrition . . . alcoholism. All I heard was *chance of survival.* I sat on Tom's sofa, frantically phoning Southwest Airlines, attempting to arrange for a last-second flight to Houston, Texas, only to discover that every single airline's flight from Nashville had departed for the evening—the last having left 30 minutes earlier. I booked the first to depart at 7 AM the following morning, July 16th. Never in my life—before or since—has a night tormented me more.

I arrived in Katy, Texas, around 11 AM and easily found the hospital that bore the same name as my daughter. I parked the rental car near the main entrance and rushed to find Intensive Care where Catherine was recovering from esophageal surgery to repair damage from intense vomiting—the first of many life-saving attempts. When I walked into the room, her appearance was so shocking to me: she was emaciated, yet her face so swollen. Her gorgeous, silky brunette hair was piled atop her head in a filthy tangled rat's nest heap—tangible evidence of her mind's darkness—and I walked up to clasp her dirty little hand. This was NOT the same person I'd last seen in my vain attempt at her birthday celebration in April when things had gone so amok.

She looked at me and barely whispered. So weak, yet she was restless . . . agitated . . . . angry. Her friend Deb was in the room. She told me Catherine wanted Colin to go get her "special bottle" (evidently her vodka). The gravity of her alcoholism was all becoming quite clear to me—how she'd turned to booze to ease the pain of her vision loss. Thinking back at that moment, I saw how it all began to come apart the day she got the diagnosis of LHON—the day she learned it wasn't "fixable." I was soon to learn—within a few hours, in fact—that she'd been consuming about a fifth of vodka per day since September 17, 2008—the day DNA finally gave us the answer.

I was standing in the hallway just outside the door talking to her brother on my cell phone, when suddenly a Code Blue was called to Catherine's room. Colin was with her. She'd become agitated. Her heart rate soared out of control. She went into cardiac arrest. Doctors, nurses, and technicians were rushing into her room. Colin came to me and we stood in the hallway together in total silence, absolute fear consuming us, as the team worked to save her—and did.

After what seemed a lifetime, we re-entered her room to find an extremely agitated Catherine with an oxygen mask on her face. She pulled at it and tried to speak, mumbling incoherently, and fought me when I attempted to soothe her. I was watching the heart monitor when I saw it begin to register another attack and shifted my glance to her face. Her eyes rolled back in her head and just as quickly the alarms sounded for another Code Blue. This time I knew it was critical. I picked up my purse, walked out the door, and stood weeping quietly as I watched through the adjacent window. When a nurse turned to see me peering through the glass, she shut the curtains on the 10 defibrillation shocks to Catherine's heart to bring her back to life.

About two hours later, Colin and I were summoned to enter what I can only describe as a scene that reminded me, oddly, of Frankenstein's bride stretched upon a cold laboratory table with life support tubes down her throat keeping the arched body of this partially nude female alive—her thick, dark hair scattered wildly above the head of the bed. I looked at my precious daughter lying there, took notice of the red machine positioned near her left shoulder that was obviously wheeled in to recharge the rhythm of her heart, and knew that my own heart was breaking. About a dozen or so professionals were still mingling around when Dr. Drtil—a heart rhythm specialist—turned to me and said, "This girl is blind. How much has she been drinking and where is she getting her alcohol?"

In a tearful, weeping confessional, Colin told of how he'd kept Catherine supplied with vodka while he traveled on his job, only because she determinedly sought to get it herself if he didn't. He told how she'd crossed heavily trafficked highways with her blind stick to go to the liquor store while he'd covertly watched from his truck and vowed he'd never put her in that desperate position again. His brokenness was confounded by the pitiful prospect of Catherine lying on that hospital bed, and I vowed I'd never hurt him more by uttering a word against him. Even Dr. Drtil put his arm around Colin and said, "We can't stand in judgment of you. You did what you thought was best."

With her doctors gathered around me, I questioned them about her chances now that these unforeseen attacks had deteriorated her condition. Ten-to-fifteen percent, I was told. "But she has *youth* on her side," they reassured me. Dr. Akhtar, another heart specialist, informed me scans revealed the alcohol had enlarged her heart and caused it to pump at only half its capacity. Her kidneys, liver, and all other vital organs were adversely affected too, and only time would tell if she'd suffered brain damage from lack of oxygen in the periods in which she had actually died. It was suggested to me that in order for Catherine to be weaned from the alcohol (generally about a three-day period) we should put her into a drug-induced coma for her body to survive the DTs.

Propofol—it had just killed Michael Jackson earlier that summer and was now the drug of choice to ease Catherine's pain and keep her in a comatose state. It was in a glass bottle and looked like milk to me. At one point, I counted 18 bags of various fluids, platelets, whole blood, and medications that were being pumped into her all at once via a pic line that had to be installed in her upper chest. She was, of course, breathing through a respirator and looked so sick, so vulnerable. Three days and nights went by in this critical state. So far, I'd never left her. I never took off my shoes. I fitfully slept on a sofa outside the Intensive Care Unit with her big fluffy stuffed bear as my pillow—it somehow brought comfort. The ICU staff always allowed me access to check on her regardless of the hour—to stroke her arms; sing to her; tell her how much I loved her. One time Colin was in the room with her cell phone in his pocket and it rang her familiar ring tone. From a deep coma, her eyes suddenly popped open in recognition of the sound and I found myself laughing. It felt so good—if only for that brief moment.

On day four of her deep slumber, the doctors and nurses determined to waken her, as statistically, by then, the alcohol should be totally out of her system and less effectual with the delirium tremens. From the moment she awoke, Catherine was irritated and anxious and angry. I had so hoped for a smile, a kind word to me for coming so far to be with her, but she was, in my opinion, still in alcohol withdrawal. I said as much to the nurses. Not possible, they said—alcohol is out of the system in 72 hours. I knew my daughter, though, and she was still in withdrawal. In her anger, she yelled at me and told me to leave her room (I was later told she asked for me not two minutes later).

One of the nurses looked at me as I dejectedly walked from the room and said: "Ms. Sandra, go get some sleep somewhere other than here. You need it. We'll take good care of her and call you if anything happens." I wrote my cell number on her white board and left, driving up and down Interstate 10 for 45 minutes looking for an affordable room—refusing to go to her house to sleep in the bed where she'd lay there since April—surrounded by vodka bottles and waste—dying.

It was 1:15 AM. My cell phone rang. I jumped up in a stupor in the strangeness of my surroundings and grabbed it too late. I saw the call had come from Christus St. Catherine Hospital. Oh, My Sweet God! I looked up the number in the directory from the night stand and called. Why hadn't I written down the direct line to ICU? Finally I reached Meka, her night nurse, who told me Catherine had "coded" a third time and had been put back into a coma to save her. She told me this third time was not as critical as the last. She said: "Go back to sleep if you can. You'll need the rest. Come back in the morning and we'll talk with you then."

At around 2 AM my cries reached out to Tom so far away in Tennessee. He had been to church without me that day to pray for Catherine. He told me to reach for the Gideon Bible in the nightstand and comfort myself with scripture before trying to sleep again, which I did. I arose at 4 AM, ate yogurt at the continental breakfast bar downstairs, walked out into the muggy July Texas heat before sunrise, and drove back to face the doctors with a huge decision for me to make.

"In order for her to ever survive outside a hospital setting, it will be necessary." That statement from Dr. Drtil was all I needed to convince me to sign the documents permitting the installation of a defibrillator/pacemaker in Catherine's heart. "Will it always be there?" I asked. Yes. The electrical rhythms of her heart were vacillating wildly and she desperately needed this device to control them.

A few days after the installation of the defibrillator, fever set in. ICU was cold to start with, but fans were brought in to blow on her in an attempt to cool her body temperature. She was shrouded in the thinnest of hospital gowns and now quite bloated all over from the many fluids being pumped into her. I felt so sorry for her, as I would see her shiver, yet I couldn't cover her with anything at all—not even a sheet. Her head began to draw to the right and I feared she would have a terrible crick in her neck whenever she awoke from this coma so I propped rolled towels beneath her head to aright the position somewhat. I would sing Moon River, watch her every breath, and pray. The fever didn't break for about 4 days.

Compression cuffs were on Catherine's legs for the entire time she was in ICU—the purpose of which were to keep blood clots from forming in the legs. Catherine's legs and feet had already suffered peripheral nerve damage and were not only numb but painful—only I never knew until then the reason being from severe alcohol consumption. The cuffs were strapped on her legs with Velcro and compressed periodically with air. I began to notice that one of her legs—the right one—was much larger than the other. It was, in fact, about twice the size of the left leg. An x-ray was done to reveal an extremely large blood clot near her groin that was causing lack of circulation in her leg. Immediate surgery was done to install a filter above the clot to catch any portion of it should it break away and move toward her heart, lungs, or brain.

Twelve long days passed with Catherine in her coma netherworld. I was always careful to keep the television on a channel with something she might enjoy, like *Malcolm in the Middle*, *The Golden Girls*, or a program of a Christian nature. I never knew what might be churning in her mind—upsetting her, perhaps. Most of my own time was spent at her bedside or in the chapel in prayer. I finally got the courage to go to her house to attend to the horrific task of tossing out bag after garbage bag of empty vodka bottles and venturing into what seemed to me the "death den" in which she'd lain for nearly three months prior in her depression. It sickened me.

I stayed for another week as she quite slowly came to reality—ordered tests having revealed no brain damage from lack of oxygen during the three Code Blues. For almost four months now Catherine had not walked. Her legs had atrophied and physical therapy was called in with a walker to help her learn the basics of reusing her legs. I'd walk with her throughout ICU and take her into the waiting room where I'd spent so many nights sleeping on the couch in the initial critical days and nights. I would gently try to reason with her about her choices once she was released, but began to sense that no matter how much I pleaded with her, she would return to drinking to block the pain of her vision loss. All I could do was give it over to GOD and hope for the best. I'd accomplished all I could.

The day I left her she was sitting on the bed in CCU where she'd spent the last 5 days at Christus St. Catherine. I was stroking her beautiful brunette hair—clean, shiny, and lovely again after 6 ½ hours of shampooing, combing and detangling. I wept openly and told her how much I loved her and begged for her to get proper help for the drinking. My month-long stay had worn on me. I needed to go.

From the window of the plane I saw a fireball sunset like none I'd ever seen—only in Texas is nature so big and grand—and prayed GOD would know the brokenness of my heart, hear my pleas, save my daughter and use her for HIS greater, mighty purpose. I gave my troubles to HIM from high in the Heavens at that moment.

I have no way of recalling when my coma ended and my very deeply drugged reality began. It wouldn't even matter for description's sake anyway. It was all just a run-on dream that was so vivid at times, with particular scenes in

101

this almost cartoon-like setting that lasted for many days. In a coma or awake, my existence was all a big hallucination. Some memories from that time are clearer than others. I can only assume that when I started murmuring, I was awake. For example, I remember how loud the tennis players in the hallway were hitting the ball back and forth and the roar it drew from the crowd. This must have been "post-coma" because I was asking for someone to please make them stop playing tennis.

Before realizing I was even in a hospital, I knew my mother was there with me. With my eyes open, I saw her blurry face—one I would always recognize and know. But even though I was just now seeing her, I knew I had been hearing her voice for quite some time. She had been saying, "Mommy's here with you," in my ear the whole time. It took forever for my brain to understand that I was in the hospital and what that meant. I was in severe pain but was too incoherent to register it. I was in flight mode and, even though incapacitated, would often try to get out of bed. In my mind these were long bizarre scenarios where I was escaping capture. When I wasn't trying to get out of bed (never successfully, and ending up in restraints, not realizing I couldn't walk), I laid there moaning in pain. I tried desperately to sleep in such agony, with the countless forms of life-support running in and out of me and all the noise it took to monitor me. Everything was chirping and beeping, and the round-the-clock tests and injections meant I got no rest.

Somehow I knew my Uncle Bern was there. He'd come from Atlanta to spend five days to support my Mom and me. I was saying the craziest, sometimes embarrassing, incoherent things to this dear respected patriarch of my family. He, like my mom, sang "Moon River" to me through his tears. Knowing how poisoned my body was from massive alcohol consumption, what I was experiencing in the way of hallucinations was more likely due to Delirium Tremens than any medications in my body, including Propofol. Even my moments of reality, like a short conversation with my mom, uncle, or Colin were clouded by visual and auditory hallucinations. The few words I could put together to communicate were almost inaudible from the abuse my vocal cords took from the feeding tube. They became strangers to me within seconds and then my whispering mumbling didn't matter anyway. I remember having to be cleaned up like an infant. In some of my crazed DT moments I pulled out my catheter not knowing what it was or even where I was.

I eventually understood that surgery had been performed on my heart. I didn't know what this meant only that it hurt. When it became safe for me I was forced to try, for just moments at a time, to sit up with my legs over the bed and eventually stand holding onto a walker. This seemed to take forever. Hardly any movement made the monitors on my weak heart go off with warning beeps. One painful step became five. I knew I had to walk if I was ever going to leave that hospital. When they moved me to CCU the staff began talking about what to do with me. My health was no longer critical, but I had been through so much no one dared to send me home. I knew some sort of alcohol treatment was imminent. Although a decision was several days to come I was told I wasn't going anywhere until I could at least walk without falling, using the walker and the bathroom on my own. I became a very motivated patient. Although the concept of time was still foreign, I knew my mom had been there quite a while and couldn't stay much longer. I wanted her to stay long enough to know where I was headed.

I was repeatedly told that if I drank again, it would kill me. The alcoholism was still fresh enough in my mind to argue this fact. I can't say that all I wanted to do was get out of there and start to drink again, but I still felt the possibility of long-term sobriety was nil. Of course I refused all treatment options provided. I was just going to go home and drink nothing for a long time—slowly merging into a life of normal, even social, drinking. The absurdity of someone who had suddenly lost their sight being sober through life was so obvious to me. What I wasn't grasping *at all* was the severity of what had just happened! My idea of returning home was as preposterous to the staff *then* as it is to me *now*. I could agree to go to inpatient alcohol treatment for a minimum required number of days, or be declared mentally incapable of caring for myself and be forced to go. Funny how, even though God had just spared my life, the state would have to force me to make the effort to turn it around!

I just wanted it all to be over. I wanted the constant bargaining between my mom, the staff, and me, to be over. Everyone kept explaining all that I had just been through and what kind of recovery it would take. I explained that this recovery would, of course, best take place where I was most comfortable—at home. They knew that I had to begin recovering from the now-proven fatal disease of alcoholism and that my body would unfortunately just have to recover along with me at a center of their choosing. Again, I never saw sobriety as a reality in my life. All I knew is that I wanted out of there, and apparently since drinking got me in there I couldn't drink like before ever again. No one seemed to understand that although I was now revived and alive, I was still blind and, therefore, just as dead as before!

I agreed to go to inpatient treatment. After being told there was a few days' waiting list, my mom packed the few things she had been living with and arranged to go home. She begged me to please, please get help, but more than anything promise never to forget the miracle that just happened and never risk my life again by drinking. The day my mother left for home I sobbed like a child being left at school on the first day. Days later I was taken by ambulance to the treatment center. My condition was more critical than I had led on at the hospital; barely able to complete the physical activity required for me to leave. I was so very sick still and used my cane to purposely isolate myself as different and unable to participate. I slept through those state required five nights. I explained to the physician upon whom my release depended that an outpatient program, near my house, where my low vision devices were, was much more suitable. I left there that blazing August day and got in Colin's truck. I realized how much people really do throw their hands up and accept a situation like alcoholism for an adult-acquired disability of this severity.

This was apparent more than ever at the intensive outpatient center I attended near my house for less than two weeks. My program was set up for me to attend eight weeks of classes for three hours a day. There were maybe six or seven other people in attendance at the same time. We shared our stories and watched videos. I couldn't see any of the videos and my story was quite unlike any others. Discussion often turned from group interaction to interrogation about what happened to me and how no one had believed what just happened.

I was still in intense physical pain. I really believed that what I was learning was how to start over with alcohol in my life (drinking wine with dinner or a beer every now and then). This was my alcoholism telling me what it wanted me to hear; I was too unique to have to get sober (I now know this is an alcoholic condition of the mind known as "terminal uniqueness"). I was dealt a terrible blow that I deserved to be tipsy through. The problem was I was physically unable to stop that tipsy. My body had just barely survived such an ordeal and nothing about its severity was clicking in my mind. I thought, if anything, I was revived so much that it would take an even longer time for my drinking to eventually have an adverse effect. The truth was, I would never have made it out of a second emergency room trip alive.

My disease was arguing in my head with the rational, functioning nourished part of my brain. I wanted to get sober to say that I could, and because I knew how much everyone pulling for me would be let down if I didn't. But I was still convinced everyone would understand about my drinking. What I had no idea of was how short-lived any "normal" drinking would be and how quickly my disease would pick up where it had left off with that insane amount of consumption. So, finally admitting defeat in my head to alcohol, I explained to the staff how terribly costly and unreliable cab transportation was. And because they wouldn't provide transportation I would have to complete my program at a later time. It was always everyone else's fault.

Alcohol truly was out of my system for several weeks. I wasn't shaking or sick during the day, but my mind still thought it was preposterous to not be able to drink and relax after another terrible day without sight. My glasses of wine with dinner became a bottle of wine during the day. And why would I drink beer? Although it is alcohol, I don't prefer the taste over liquor. So then, flavored vodka soon returned. Then came the very cheap variety. I was not alone much anymore so I drank secretly, but knew it was obvious. I lied on the phone about my drinking to everyone who called to check on me after the hospital stay.

I even got involved, again, with DARS. They sent someone to my home for beginning lessons with assistive software on the PC they also provided for me. Even though I was visually impaired, I somehow thought my instructor wouldn't know I was drunk because he was blind! I was so hooked I did not care. I had to feel the hot stream of vodka going down my throat before beginning any task like talking on the phone or attempting to listen to computer instructions. The DTs were back when alcohol left my system for more than a half day. Colin took me to Moody Gardens in Galveston one day. I honestly thought, if I tried, I could make it through the day sober. I would not bring any booze with me and I would make myself do it. Only two hours into our day I tearfully admitted that he had to drive me to the liquor store so I could fill up a water bottle for the day.

I denied all drinking to my mom, but I think she knew. I knew I was spiraling downward and knew that this end meant death. But instead of begging for an end this time I was stuck in an alcoholic purgatory with no way out. I went home to Tennessee for Thanksgiving—three months after my release from the hospital. I was badly, physically addicted like before, and brought several bottles in my suitcase to make it through the trip. My mom found these and, out of terror for what she had seen just a few months before, poured every drop down the sink.

I lost it in a full-blown panic attack when I found them gone. I explained to her how much I was drinking again and that I simply could not go through the withdrawals. She phoned the hospital and they did suggest that it was unsafe to cut me off entirely. I'll never forget telling the person on the other end that she had to ask them these questions although she was "so fuming mad" she could scream at me. How pathetic, I thought. It being Thanksgiving, and with the liquor stores closed, my poor mom had to make phone calls to find even a single friend with liquor she could come pick up to give me so I could get through dinner and the next morning. There was and never had been anything to drink in my mom's house. Just like my being affected by LHON is an anomaly in my family so is my drinking.

On schedule, with the effects of the last sip from that begged-for bottle waning, the withdrawals started. Mom took me to Middle Tennessee Medical Center in Murfreesboro, Tennessee. My anxiety and shakes soared while waiting in the emergency room all day waiting for various tests to return back abnormal, requiring my admittance. I was there to detoxify and heal for eight days. My family from my dad's side came to visit since I was now in Tennessee. No one knew what to really say: it's as if everyone was coming to pity what was left of the girl for whose loss they now grieved. My mom tried desperately to get me to get admitted in inpatient alcohol treatment while I was home, but since I was on Medicaid in Texas, this would have to wait until I got back.

With sad and defeated hugs, and the promise of my immediate check-in for help made, I left for Texas again. I was so relieved to learn that the healthcare system would pay for alcoholism treatment. The problem was the long, unavoidable waiting list, for a bed at a facility. There was no actual waiting list, as spots were given on a first-come-first-served basis (if available at all) when calling at 7 AM every morning. The bureaucracy and red tape for this state-funded institution made this process so exasperating. I was still seeing my therapist, infrequently, but I had admitted to her that I need inpatient treatment but couldn't stop drinking while waiting. She said they would probably understand and to keep calling every morning. I was placed on hold every morning at 7 AM and by 8 o'clock, sometimes before someone even came back on the line to say there was nothing, I was beaten. The nausea, anxiety and downright mental obsession had won and I was drunk.

I knew that my second appointment in the LHON clinical study in Miami was to be December 9th, now just a week away. It looked as though I would be in attendance and not in an inpatient treatment facility. I know now that God was planning things in His perfect timing. I wouldn't get at the real emotional issues for my drinking until almost the last day of that damned year, 2009. Knowing I couldn't physically make it through a trip to Miami in my condition—and definitely not succeed as a participant in any study—I checked myself into an emergency detox facility, where I stayed drugged through the DTs for five days and nights only to come out sober and get on a plane to Miami.

Jeff again went with me, and this time I was able to get through the long day of testing with ease. I was so busy focusing, mentally and physically with my eyes, test after test on my sight during that all-day appointment that I never entertained the thought of continuing sobriety. I just wanted to get through that day, followed by an early evening plane ride home. Again I was physically sober; not a drop of alcohol in my body to make me crave more of it or make decisions about drinking it. What I was experiencing instead was a complete mental obsession for alcohol run riot.

As I saw the beverage cart being pushed up the aisle my mind was running a mile a minute. It was saying two things that I believed: I deserved a drink after completing that hard day and that I was waiting for room in a treatment facility anyway. I thought if I could just get off the plane, though, I would return home where there was no alcohol and no one to buy it for me and I would be fine. I waited until we almost began the final descent until I went to the back, found the figure of a person I assumed could help me, and ordered two airline bottles of Jack Daniels, one for me and one for Jeff. Because, hey, it wasn't vodka and Jeff was going home to Tennessee, so I thought we could celebrate with Tennessee whiskey! This baffling disease seemed to reward me for giving into it because the flight attendant gave us two bottles each and didn't charge anything. The next day, with Jeff gone, and me back in Houston, my insane mind lost the battle with alcohol once again—this time scrounging up cab fare only to ride in the back seat to the store silent with nausea and panic tearing me up from that comparably little amount I'd drunk the night before.

I learned in recovery that insanity is repeating the same mistake over and over again and expecting different results. Not only was I admittedly insane on December 10th, 2009, I was also a walking dead person. I knew I would die, but thought I was physically revived enough to last for some time—maybe long enough to get the help that everyone including myself was so desperately waiting for. Knowing I was facing imminent death, and having to drink alcohol constantly to make my mind and body function, was the point at which I had my rock bottom. This was my pitiful and incomprehensible demoralization that most true alcoholics so desperately need to reach the humility required for change.

Colin came to Houston to get me to go with him to San Antonio to spend Christmas with his family. They were my family away from home for the years I was in Texas. I had no choice but to tell him I was going to have to drink until I got the answer I hoped for on the other end of the phone every morning: yes, there is a bed at a facility. If he wasn't going to supply me with vodka while we were at his parents, I would stay home alone and get cab rides over Christmas. Poor Colin, of course he took me with him to San Antonio where on December 29th the news came that I could enter treatment that day in Houston if I hurried from San Antonio three hours away. I knew this would be a 28-day stay. Phoning home, leaving messages, crying and telling anyone who answered that I'd be gone, I drank my last drop to this day in Colin's truck, as he pulled up to the condemned looking house that is now a treatment facility.

I went in that place humiliated, defeated, and literally dying for help. I explained that I couldn't see. This wasn't a problem—at least not yet—because all I needed to know was how to feel my way to the bathroom. The first order of business in this non-medical facility was to knock me out and let me sleep it off. It was hell and my whole body hurt. As a side note, I discovered six months later at a check-up appointment with a cardiologist who reads my pacemaker/defibrillator activity via print out, that my heart began palpitating wildly on January 1, 2010, three days into my stay. My mom and I are so thankful to God for guiding her in the decision to have it placed in my chest those months before. Only He knew that I would need it to help me stay alive in order to do what I'd failed to do before—surrender my will to Him. All of my resistance to His plan, His work in my life, whatever the reason, had left myself open for complete denial, depression and ultimate wish for death if I couldn't have my sight. Fighting so hard against the psychological pain of my sight loss had left me badly physically addicted to alcohol, and now the pain of drinking and surviving in such a condition became greater than the idea of pushing through the initial physical withdrawal and finally letting go and letting God take over.

But God had mercy on me yet again. He had already saved my life three times in the hospital and now He was there again. He spared me the DTs while withdrawing during those first few days at Houston's Volunteers of America (VOA) where I sobered up and successfully completed treatment despite the reading/writing curriculum for therapy. This is where I began my constant prayer for guidance in every move (a must for a white-knuckled alcoholic) took over and saved me. I refused to be terminally unique anymore—letting my disability keep me from doing the work that real sobriety requires and, therefore, not getting better because I "couldn't." When I felt well enough to fight my disability and not drown in it for once, I worked out a system with the staff so I could complete assignments like everyone else.

The mere mention of a possible Americans with Disabilities Act violation of my rights to proper medical care really helped expedite the outline for a therapy plan. I voice recorded and turned in on tape the same required assignments for the other thirty or so female inmates. When they had to read essays about their actions and consequences, I did just as well, taking my time through tears and squinting at my black marker scrawled and scrambled pages (my 20 to their 3, but the same amount of words). I wasn't the misfit in the

109

treatment facility that my blindness made me in the world outside. Everyone was especially touched by my story and how the disease of addiction really crosses all lines among people. The other girls said how brave and inspiring I was. I couldn't believe it. Never did I think these would be the first times of so many to come that I would hear those same words.

I'll never forget how cold that barely heated house was the whole month of January or how desperate the circumstances under which I had to get sober. I wore donated clothes, ate donated food, and did daily chores like everyone else there. I was deloused, TB tested, bussed and strip-searched in and out of the home and allowed 10 minutes on the phone per day—only after eight days of strict rehabilitation, just like everyone else. But *unlike* them I was *there on my own accord*. This was a court appointed Rehab facility and I was the only one who *voluntarily chose to be there*. I desperately wanted and needed to get this help and make this work—finally. I sincerely believe that this VOA house, in shambles, and freezing, made for the tough lesson in humility and feeling of "last hope" that I needed for real change. I never, ever want to go back. I'd found myself scraping the bottom of life, starting over with nothing but regret and waning faith in myself. LHON began my journey of healing that took me to the depths of despair and back into a life of faith in God, myself, and in humanity.

I don't know about the other girls, but the cold ego-breaking, laborious, and emotionally excruciating tough love of VOA stuck with me. By the Grace of God, I have never returned to it or any other similar facility and, one day at a time, I never will. Some girls were in there to pay their debt for probation violation and to return to incarceration, if not success at completing the program. I saw some go back to jail directly from there. Some were due to be released with uncertainty regarding the reconnection of family relations. My loved ones were so far away that Colin came to the required "family therapy" sessions on weekends. We both knew I'd be heading home to Tennessee to be with my family—sober and ready to face life anew. We were especially weepy for my sighted life and what happened because of its loss that we'd both experienced so helplessly together. I left that facility and returned home to Tennessee on February 8, 2010, to face the challenge posed upon every alcoholic deserving sobriety—learning to accept life on life's terms.

Yes, I was still newly blind and no, it still wasn't fair. Same set of circumstances as right after my hospital stay. But this time I would fight—not against the reality of my disability, but for life! I would fight for my own chance at normalcy by rebuilding and starting over with proper tools in place. This time I knew and felt spring was just around the corner and I would come back to life and blossom and flourish in sync with it. In my heart, I felt it would be a time of rebirth—unlike when I gave up altogether the same time a year before; or when my view of life began to disappear the spring before that. I would no longer cry over not seeing landscapes or the written word. I would create my own positive, upbeat environment, involve myself daily in recovery, and surround myself with loved ones. I would begin to journal, document, and process what had happened to me so as to be helpful to others.

When I returned home to Tennessee, my loving family and I celebrated Christmas that had waited for me. With the house still decorated in February, we had a warm celebration of hope and love like none other. I thought about my other inmates at VOA and wondered if their receptions at home would be as joyful as mine. There's never been a moment I've failed to think of my great fortune in having such support from my family.

My 30th year and a new decade ushered in *sober* that spring—filled with renewed hope and personal growth. I felt great—physically, spiritually, mentally. I began computer-training classes that same week provided by Tennessee Vocational Rehabilitation. Learning and retention was easy for me with a clear mind and optimism for disability training. I was told in treatment that as hard as I had worked to get liquor *despite* my disability, I'd need to work twice as hard to fight for my turn-around out of disability-blamed despair and, consequently, my next drink. I did and quickly found that I wasn't just a *participant* in life again; God had not only left my brain fully functioning, He'd blessed me with drive and the ability to quickly learn. He engulfed me in His love and blessings beyond my imagination. I found open, honest help and love in a perfectly placed home group for my Program of Sobriety. All I had to do was tell members where I lived, that I needed help and I couldn't see. Every audio material necessary to work the program, and anything else I needed, was quickly and eagerly provided to me. I was given rides to and from meetings anytime I needed. Looking back, this placement of me with them was surely God doing for me what I could not do for myself.

Overdue amends were made to family and loved ones who had pulled for me despite my resistance in the past. My profuse apologies were always met with the same understanding reply—that no one really knows how they would handle a similar situation until they are placed in it. My family has been nothing but ecstatic to have me whole and back in their lives. They are the first on my thankful-list each day. The best way I know to make up for the insane amount of stress I placed on my mom is to try every day to live up to the potential of her prayers. I want to live the life and fulfill the purpose that she begged God for in sparing my life when I was so critically ill.

In May of 2010, an echogram revealed that less than a year after it had repeatedly stopped (and close to forever), my heart is completely healthy. Blood tests came back normal, revealing a healthy liver. On 15 July 2010 (a year to the day after I nearly died), Mom and I returned to the ICU staff at Christus St. Catherine Hospital in Katy, Texas, to thank them for saving my life and show them, in person, how valuable their efforts are in life-saving. There were hardly any dry eyes in the place! They simply couldn't believe it was me! I also saw my therapist who had heard me wail over one loss after another for a full year. She couldn't stop beaming as I showed off the healthy me I wanted so badly for her to know was beneath all those tears.

As my growth extended beyond myself, I became involved within the disabled community by joining the Tennessee Council for the Blind. At their July convention that year, I was awarded a Braillewriter, for my determination and inspiration to learn Braille (which is a great expense cut from my upcoming and imminent task of learning it). Knowing that others who have lived without sight most, if not all, of their lives found my story unimaginably difficult and inspiring-enough to award me with valuable tools to help me along has been one of my proudest moments.

Also, that same summer, I saw my Uncle Bern for the first time since he saw me near death in the hospital. All it took was one look at me to know I was back and full of life. I told my father (graveside with my uncle) that I knew he was proud of me in Heaven. I know he's aware of what happened to his daughter and must wish he could have been here to tell me it's going to be okay; I assured him that finally it was.

As a way of transitioning back into the world of work, I spent four and a half months completing computer classes and began to realize technology was no longer obsolete to me. I was so fortunate to have been assigned an instructor from the Tennessee Disability Coalition (TDC) who was supportive, and who believed in my potential to achieve and reach beyond any self-imposed limitations. During her last week of training with me, she informed me of a job opening within that same non-profit organization. Five short months after first walking into the TDC building—feeling nervous, wary, not yet sure of myself—I walked out a temporary employee as an organizer to rally the disability vote in the upcoming mid-term election. This was another God-given, proud moment of my life. My prayers for guidance had been answered and it looked as though my pleas for purpose were next to come.

This job led me to speak at a retirement home meeting for residents adjusting to their new blindness. They responded so positively to me, that I alone chaired their next meeting and, again, felt how powerful supporting and helping others can be. I began to feel the genuine need to advocate for others. I was already sharing my experience, strength, and hope with other alcoholics so that they might benefit in their quest for recovery. How could I do the same with my disability? The job ended with the election and everyone praised my efforts. At a wrap party to celebrate a job-well-done by all of the organizers, we were asked to share with Coalition staffers an unforgettable experience we'd had while on the team. More than once I heard from others that they were inspired by working with me. I had found a place in which I could not only "make it" but excel in advocacy.

Having done so years before, but now with newfound meaning and with great support, I began to study the very next week for the Law School Admissions Test (LSAT) in hope of possible acceptance to law school. Vocational Rehabilitation provided me with twelve weeks of tutoring prior to the 12 February 2011 test date. While in the midst of intense study (29 December 2010), I celebrated one year of sobriety—a year to the day from that sad, helpless, entry into Volunteers of America. On the day of the administration of the LSAT, I was met with many testing irregularities at Vanderbilt University, prompting me to want to fight even harder for those like me—to make equitable accommodations for the disabled.

Even though I was testing *completely orally* against the best of circumstances, I still achieved a high score on the LSAT and was accepted to law school to begin the 2011 Fall Term—my childhood dream finally realized! In retrospect, I can honestly say that LHON took away my sight to give me *insight*. It brought me through the worst time of my life—the greatest of despair and nearly took my life—and through God's intervention, brought me back whole again. I am not giving up hope for sight restoration, but in the meantime, I am dedicating my life to disability advocacy. I want to earn my Jurisprudence Degree in order to give credibility to my voice that will be heard by many to bring about *change*.

Catherine's note: in the 15 months that have passed since writing this chapter, amazing things have happened in my life. I grew from being a ball of nerves on the verge of tears when I began law school to a member of the Dean's List who loves class and camaraderie. I was recognized for my merits by the American Council of the Blind, the Tennessee Council of the Blind, and the Council for Citizens with Low Vision International, who each awarded me a scholarship. I am now in my second year and determined, more than ever, to be an effective advocate. I look forward to celebrating three years of sobriety on December 29, 2012, God willing and one day at a time.

Catherine Knight

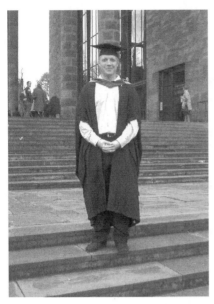
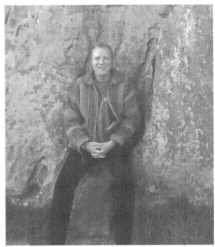

A Taste of Emotions by David Rosser

The feel of autumn was in the air, the wind had cooled and the aroma of the plants had a more earthy smell. Soon my job as a lifeguard working at an outdoor swimming pool would be coming to an end. What was I going to do with my life? I was just 20 years old.

Since leaving school at 16 I had worked as a car mechanic, following career advise from my mother and her mantra of, "You will never be out of work if you have a trade." But hey ho, it wasn't for me so I stuck it out for my three long years apprenticeship, got my papers after qualifying and left, never to return to car mechanics again, apart from a number of restoration projects for myself on classic cars with Triumph GT6's and Spitfires being my passion.

My career change was greatly influenced by my best friend Lewis who also had decided to do an apprenticeship but in the building trade, but shortly after qualifying went to work as a lifeguard and looked so happy since making the transition in jobs. He told me a course was coming up which would enable me to qualify as a lifeguard. I had swam competitively in my younger days and passed the course easily and had lots of fun on the way. My first job lifeguarding was at an outdoor water park in the summer near my home. It was a summer of endless parties, women, constant laughter, and fun.

The weather was getting colder as the summer was coming to an end. Lewis and I decided to get jobs at a local holiday camp as lifeguards working indoors for the winter—let the parties continue. At the beginning of the following summer I got a job at another holiday camp and was given the grand title of head lifeguard. There, I made friends that would stay with me to this day.

I was getting into this lifestyle of working outdoors for the summer and fancied spending the winter somewhere hot abroad. I noticed a job in the local paper for selling timeshares in Tenerife, one of the Canary Islands which is off the coast of Africa and which is hot all year. I applied for the job and had an interview, but I never heard anything else. My job finished as a lifeguard and I threw caution to the wind, booked a flight and just went out to Tenerife, where the company I had the interview in England was based.

I reached Tenerife Airport, picked up my bags, and went through immigration. However just as I was leaving the airport and much to my surprise and to the surprise of the guy that held the interviews for selling timeshare, we bumped into each other. I said hello and he asked what are you doing here. I said I've come to sell timeshare and he said you've got yourself a job. After a few months I decided it wasn't for me: maybe it was the daily lies of no, it's not timeshare sir/madam, and I got another job outside a bar promoting the bar/nightclub.

The first night I clicked with an English guy called Sean who was also doing the same job as me and who was mad as a hatter and had lived in Holland. We decided to go back to Holland for a two-week holiday and I ended up spending a year of my life in Holland. I worked hard and partied hard. Well, I was 21 and had boundless energy. When no work was around we would just nip to Germany and pick up bits here and there. The norm was to go out on a Friday and party like crazy until Monday, often going to work Monday morning after not sleeping all weekend. I would spend the week recovering before doing it all again. After a year it was becoming all too much so I decided to make the sensible decision and head back to England for a summer around the swimming pool as a lifeguard.

116

The company I had previously worked for welcomed me back with open arms and it was great to see so many familiar faces: it was like one big family. Whilst out one night with my work colleagues I met a woman, Claire, and we fell madly in love with each other. Hey, this wasn't meant to happen; however, she had a profound impact on me and would have an incredible influence on my perception of life in the future. Claire loved my tales of travelling and one day asked if I would go travelling with her at the end of the summer. Bonus: more winter sun and a beautiful woman to join me, but the truth was that I was honoured by her offer and Claire was starting to melt my macho male ego, which was only a good thing.

Claire and I had a very enriching relationship, often trying new activities as we learned to scuba dive amongst many other things, and a very memorable parachute jump that went not quite to plan. We had trained for 3 days for the parachute jump and four of us went up in a light aircraft. When we were 4,500 feet up, we had to click a line to the inside of the aircraft (this was so that all we had to do is jump and the static line attached to the plane would open the chute automatically). Three people jumped prior to me and then I walked sideways onto the wing and proceeded to jump off. Only seconds before this the instructor had said don't worry, nothing ever goes wrong (Shock, horror, I thought: what a stupid thing to say, the perfect recipe for something to go wrong).

So there I was falling through the air and I decided to look up like they teach you in training to check that the chute has opened and the lines are as they should be. Well, to my disbelief, only half the chute at best had opened and all the lines were tangled. Apparently they could hear my swearing from the ground: it's not like you can say stop the ride, I want to get off. I thought hard and quick, saying "think." I think to myself, weighing the options. It was a case of do I cut away where I pull a cord to release the parachute, then free fall (not that we had done free fall parachuting in training), and then pull the reserve parachute. Would that maybe work, my internal dialogue continued.

The alternative, which I chose, was to put my arms out in a crucified position, look up to see which way the cords were tangled and spin around like a possessed man fighting for his life. Eventually as the ground got closer and people's eyes on the ground got bigger, the cords untwisted and the chute fully inflated. Shortly afterwards I landed and the instructor said calmly, the chute must have been badly packed. I then proceeded to laugh more from a feeling of euphoria and said, "Badly fucking packed." One day I will do another parachute jump and enjoy the experience.

The plans for travelling were made and we decided to go to London for the weekend and book the trip whilst we were there. At the end of the summer we flew from London to Bali in Indonesia, then flew into Melbourne, Australia. We then flew out of Brisbane to Singapore, making our way over land to Malaysia. We made our way into Thailand and flew out of Bangkok to London eight months later, so hopefully I could get my summer job back as a lifeguard. The trip was full of wonderful, positive experiences apart from one time when I was bitten by a stingray in Southern Thailand on a remote island with no roads, just dirt tracks, miles from anywhere and huts on the beach with no electricity and where some days you just didn't see people.

The sea was like a hot bath and Claire and I were probably up to our chests, having fun messing around when something bit me in my foot. "Shit," I shouted to Claire, "something's just bitten me." She took off for the beach faster than an Olympic swimmer closely followed by me. Within seconds I could feel something that can only be described as a line of pain, which was poison travelling up the vein in my leg and when it got to my hip I lost all sensation and function in my legs. By this point I was under the water unable to use my legs and had to make the 20 metres to the beach just with my arms.

Eventually I made it to the beach, having to pull myself up the beach with my arms as my legs just didn't work. My brain raced away with thoughts of sea snakes before a woman standing on a nearby cliff top shouted, "You've been bitten by a stingray; it's their breading season." This was somewhat embarrassing as I had no clothes on at the time, but then I thought thank God for that, at least it wasn't a sea snake; as I was in the middle of nowhere and it was probably hours if not a considerable distance more to the nearest hospital.

If the poison had travelled any further up my body then I would have been in big trouble. The gods were smiling on me that day. Minutes later the woman appeared next to me and said she was a nurse in Germany and told me to take these tablets, which were pain killers. I promptly took the pain killers, almost crying in pain, and within half an hour—which seemed like forever—the pain subsided to a manageable level. I was left with two small cuts in the bottom of my foot where the stingray had bitten me. The next day I was back in the water swimming around snorkeling, but much more cautious of the sea life.

On returning to England I went back to working as a lifeguard and Claire became very career focused and got a job with the local council. Her parents were having relationship problems which hit Claire hard. I was also being non-committal in the relationship as Claire wanted us to live together, but I felt I was too young and also enjoyed my care-free life. We ended up seeing less and less of each other, and eventually we split. I was devastated and it took me a long time to bounce back. The only positive of Claire and I splitting was that I went on a spiritual journey—which I am still on—and it shaped my life forever. It would be my salvation when I lost my eye sight and had major health problems.

After Claire and I split I seemed to lose focus and direction in life, trying many different types of jobs and not wanting to commit to a long-term relationship with any woman I met. Quite by chance I met a spiritual teacher called Bernie Prior who is a Self-realized teacher, whose life is entirely devoted to the awakening of all, calling for the full and uncompromised living of One's True Self. Without a shadow of doubt Bernie and his teachings changed my view on life and the world as I know it today in such a profound and positive way. At times my life became incredibly difficult with much pain and suffering, but I know now that it was like a shedding of my past to become the man I am today: a deeper, loving, caring, sensitive being living his spirituality and truth as a way of life.

I took part in many of Bernie's healing courses and retreats. The healing became known as The Form-Reality Practice, a profound vehicle of transformation for true evolutionary living, and is the principal practice of the teaching.

I decided to do some academic studying and achieved a number of qualifications in various subjects. Following a meeting with a career advisor, it was decided that I wanted to pursue a career in Occupational Therapy and have a career. Now I had some direction in my life; this was great.

Following an eight week intense healing course with Bernie, I then woke up one morning following some profound dreams and I decided that I needed to go to India to find myself. My family and some of my friends thought I was mad, but those who truly know me knew otherwise. It all felt so right, and within two weeks I was in India. I balanced my spiritual journey, having met some incredibly spiritual teachers, with some parties in Goa and some trekking in Nepal. I returned home to England a year later, considerably lighter in weight, but as a deeper spiritual person with a million more questions about life than when I had left.

I managed to achieve a place at University studying Occupational Therapy and my life seemed to have more direction. The first year passed with a blink of the eye and as I was starting the second year, I decided to do some nursing work to help with the finances. I signed up with a nursing agency and had a phone call asking if I could cover a shift at a nursing home one day. I arrived at the door and had my photo identification badge ready and was greeted by the most amazingly beautiful and tall, dark haired woman who took one look at me and ran off. A guy then came to the door and when I asked who that was, he replied, "Oh, that's just Jo."

It was like someone had switched a very bright light on and hooked me up to the power grid. In what can only be described as love at first sight, I knew that one day Jo and I would have children (Aurora and Athena) together. I later learned that when Jo first saw me, she was totally overcome with emotions and had a similar experience to myself. Jo says that our worlds collided with so much energy, emotion, and love of a truly deep connection that really it was just love at first sight.

We started dating and towards the end of my last year at University I asked Jo if she wanted to move to Torquay, a different part of England near the sea where I had lived before I had gone to University and she agreed; I was blown away. Life was good, in fact it was great. I had a month to go before I finished University and would be qualifying as an Occupational Therapist. I had bought a nice, fast car, a weakness of mine along with fast motorbikes, but the bike could wait until I had a job. Now I had to sort out somewhere for us to live.

I decided to go home for a long weekend to see my mates and look for somewhere to live after finishing University. Whilst home I picked my friend Lewis up and took him for a drive in my new car. We were at the traffic light waiting for it to turn green near the sea and I said the sea mist is bad today. He replied, "Sea mist, what sea mist?" The light turned green and I hit the accelerator hard, leaving a boy racer in the car next to me standing.

I stopped off at a newsagent and picked up a local paper to look for somewhere to live. I managed to find a couple of possibilities of accommodation in the paper and agreed to view them the following week with Jo. One of the flats was being renovated and it turned out that the landlord was someone that I had worked with and he promised me that it would be completed in time, and so it was agreed we were to move in a month later.

I had finished my final exam at University and just had the presentation to do about my Dissertation. That wasn't a problem as I enjoyed presentations greatly and then Jo and I could move to Torquay. I was feeling exhausted as I had been studying hard, partying hard, and also had to do paid work over the last three years. I felt like I had constant flu: my body ached and my eyes felt constantly tired. I was looking forward to moving back home by the sea and to taking a few weeks out on the beach to recharge my batteries. Burning the candle at both ends was starting to have its toll.

Jo's brother was a courier driver and he agreed to move all the furniture and our belongings down to Torquay, as he had managed to get a delivery job down that way. I felt constantly stressed for some reason, which was unlike me, and I received a phone call to say that the flat would not be ready for another month. My mother agreed that we could live with her temporarily and that we could store all the furniture at her home. It was a good job. She had a big house, but it was going to be challenging living at home again.

The day came to move all the belongings down and I followed the van in my car. For some reason my right eye kept twitching and driving in the dark seemed more difficult than usual. Other cars' headlights seemed brighter than normal, but we made it to Torquay. The following morning I offered to give Jo's brother a lift to his courier job some distance away and on the way back I had to ask him to drive my car as my eyes became so tired it was like I couldn't keep them open.

I needed a few weeks to recharge my batteries badly. In the following days my sight became blurred or maybe somewhat fuzzy and I put it down to maybe needing glasses and I made an appointment at a local opticians. I drove to the opticians and went through the usual process: can you read the letters on the board? But I couldn't read lower than the third line down. The optician said he would be back in a moment and left the room. He returned some time later and said that I had to go straight to the hospital eye department as there was something wrong with my eyes but he did not know what. I got back in the car and then drove to the hospital. Little did I know that would be my last real car journey I was to drive alone?

On arriving at the eye department they took my name and all my details and very shortly I was taken into a room by a consultant, Mr. Charlie James, a true gentleman who made the whole difficult, painful experience easier due to his caring and compassionate nature. He checked my eyes, took my ocular pressure, and then I went and had a horrible field test, which in the future I would have to do time and time again and would come to hate with a passion.

I was then asked to wait before I was seen again by the consultant who was honest and said they were unsure what was causing the problem. He wanted to run further tests, take pictures of my eyes, and give me a CT scan and an MRI scan as soon as possible. My brain raced as during my Occupational Therapy training I had worked in Palliative Care and the horrible thought of a brain tumour or something nasty crossed my mind.

My father and Jo met me at the eye department reception. I kept the thoughts of a brain tumour to myself. The receptionist said take care as we left. I could hear the heaviness in her voice: she might as well have said poor bastard. Later I would learn how to read incredible amounts of information in people's voices, which I call the frequency of the voice which is a richness of information and enables me to know if I can trust a person, know if they are lying and hear a range of emotions, which would become useful when I was to meet my Rehabilitation Officer from hell later.

My dad drove my car home and I was so glad to be with Jo, and I tried to understand what was going on. The next day I returned to the eye department with Jo and they injected some dye into my body which turned my skin orange. Apparently this was to make everything more visible in the eye, and they promptly took lots and lots of photos. I was given drops for my eyes as I had glaucoma and the ocular pressure was very high. I thought, "What the hell is glaucoma?" I learned that a distant family member had suffered with glaucoma, but I was the first to have anything like this.

Over the coming days it's like my body shut down, or went into free fall mode, as the shock of what was going on hit me. I felt like death warmed up. I was 31 years old; it was my favourite time of year, the summer, well the end of the summer, August 2003. But I was invincible; strong, fit, and healthy; even bullet proof; the world was my oyster. I had just qualified from University as an Occupational Therapist, something I had dreamed of and worked hard towards for many years. I had found my soul mate and was going to be living with her. I was at the start of a new chapter in my life, on the crest of a wave, but life isn't a shopping list of wants and needs and I was on a different chapter in God's big plan.

My mind struggled to keep up with my body, as for the first time in my life I was not in control of what was going on. It took me back to the time I had jumped out of a plane and my parachute didn't open properly. This was a frightening, yet humbling experience and I even thought was I going to die. Would I survive this, as I felt so ill? I had to embrace the experience and look at it through my spiritual eyes. There was no way I was going to run from this and have it haunt me for years: I had to deal with whatever came up for me. For this I thank all the people I have cared for in Palliative Care who unknowingly taught me so much and little did I know that I would be my own Occupational Therapist so quickly after qualifying. At times through great pain and suffering came moments of deep peace and calmness, which was extraordinarily profound and spiritual.

I developed tremors, muscle weakness, and had no energy to even eat. It was a struggle to make it to the toilet; in fact, even going to the toilet was exhausting and would wipe my energy levels out for hours. My doctor put me on Fortisip, an energy/meal replacement drink for the elderly or people who are very ill, which helped greatly. However, I just didn't have any energy to do anything and often spent days in bed just sleeping.

I developed an allergy to most chemicals: bleach, hairspray, and perfumes to name a few. The result of being in the same space as these chemicals was that my body would go into shock, I would start sweating profusely, and a pressure would build in my body. Once this started I had to sit or lie down and control my breath until the feeling passed, as my heart beat so fast it sounded like a big base drum. Some years later I learned that my body's immune system was so low that the chemicals were causing me to have anaphylactic shocks.

I went for the MRI and CT scans and on both occasions my consultant was there and told me instantly all was clear. I said to him I know what you were thinking: Cancer. He just said its all clear, but we have more tests to do. The tests ticked the boxes off the long list of what it could be, but we still didn't know what it was. The waves of tiredness still crashed hard on my body and I had this constant all over body pain; I felt like I had been beaten up badly.

For weeks I continued to wake up thinking I could see, hoping that my sight would return. Then I would open my eyes to see that it had not and the reality of what happened kicked in. I started getting hallucinations and was told by the consultant that this was due to the brain being starved of sensory information. I later learned this was called Charles Bonnet Syndrome and I would give talks and presentations on the subject later whilst working. The hallucinations went on for months and reminded me of my long weekends in Holland using LSD, which in a strange way helped with managing the symptoms. Jo would often say, "Dave, stop playing with them (the hallucinations)," and we would laugh. At times they were intense; they would not even go away when I closed my eyes, and felt very real to me. It was like being on mind altering drugs for weeks on end: exhausting.

A so called top specialist in Neurology had heard about me and wanted to see me. He had a monthly clinic at my local hospital and it was agreed that I would meet him. On meeting him with Jo, I took an instant dislike to him. His bed side manner was terrible and he had little or no people skills. He spent the whole time talking to Jo about me as if I was invisible; there was no point in me being there. But I decided to go to his hospital ward as it specialized in Neurology and I wanted to know what was the matter with me as the not knowing was becoming irritating to say the least.

A bed was booked and within two weeks I was down there for two days. My dad drove me and Jo came too. The hospital was massive and my ward was in a tall block which specialized in neurological conditions and was to be my new home for the next two days where I would be prodded and poked.

The evening meal was soup, bread roll, and ice cream as they had run out of food. Due to my poor eye sight and the ward being high up I said to someone, "What's that red blur in the distance?" to which I was told Kentucky Fried Chicken. Yummy I thought, due to my health I had just burned up calories, and soup and ice cream just didn't hit the spot.

I told the nurse I had to go outside to make a phone call and made a bee line for the red blur in the distance which I knew was Kentucky Fried Chicken. Ah, my first trip out alone as a visually impaired person. It was hell. I don't know how I made it there: dodging speeding cars or what seemed like speeding cars, falling over walls, even counting my money out or how I made it back as I had no red blur to follow, but it was hard work and detracted from the enjoyment of the food. On returning to the ward the nurse was not happy and asked where I had been, to which I said to make a phone call. She replied you've been gone over an hour. Well, it was a long phone call I chuckled, but I'm sure she knew where I had been.

In the evening the consultant visited and she said that she wanted to do a lumbar puncture the next day to ascertain if I had Multiple Sclerosis and obtain crucial information from the spinal fluid, to which I agreed. All the patients on the ward were great, we all got on, but the night before my lumbar puncture I could feel myself getting more nervous. There was a lad in the corner who was only 20 and had a brain aneurism and was as nervous and anxious as me. His distraction was the TV, but with my eye sight, seeing the TV was hard work, so I didn't put it on.

The constant laughing, joking, and generally loud talking of the nurses drove me up the wall. By around 2am I asked them if they could keep the noise down and again at 3am, but they just carried on like they were having the time of their lives. Well, I thought mischievously, if they won't shut up then I'll take myself somewhere else. I jumped out of bed, took off the pillows, duvet, and sheet and walked past the nurses' station. They all stopped talking and asked where I was going, to which I replied somewhere where I can sleep in peace.

I walked off the ward and somewhere down the corridor I found an empty bed, made it up, and went to sleep. Sometime later I was awoken by a security guard who said that I would have to go back to the ward. I said only when you tell the nurses to shut up as I can't get any sleep, to which he agreed. He went off and read them the riot act: I bet that involved a lot of paperwork. We both went back to the ward and the nurses very kindly made my bed back up. I went to sleep and awoke in the morning with a dreaded feeling of the lumber puncture.

I knew what the procedure was; having worked in the medical profession, but at this point a little knowledge was a dangerous thing as my brain ran away with itself. The consultant introduced herself and her senior before starting the lumber puncture. God, it was painful and after lots of grunts and groans from the consultant she was ordered to move over by her senior consultant who finished the lumbar puncture. To this day I still struggle with a painful lumbar region which is only helped by daily core stability exercises.

Later that afternoon the consultant came and apologized for having two left hands and causing me so much pain. I asked her how many lumbar punctures she had done before to which she said I was her second. Maybe that was a question I should have asked before. Having just trained I had some sympathy for her, as there had been many patients which had agreed to let me loose on them. It's how you learn in the medical profession I suppose. I felt like I had been run over by a steam roller and when Jo turned up on the ward later and gave me a hug that afternoon I cried. I had never missed her so much in all my life.

I returned to the hospital twice more after that, once for them to put wires on my eyes to ascertain if information was getting to my brain from my eye, along the optic nerve, whilst looking at a screen with flashing checkers boards and different images. Another time they hooked my brain up to a computer to see if the brain waves were functioning correctly, but I was so exhausted I just kept falling asleep and rather embarrassingly they had to keep waking me up during the assessment. That was another couple of boxes ticked off; I never did find out if they found my brain.

On returning to my ophthalmologist he reported that the ocular pressure was reduced greatly and that I only needed to apply eye drops in the evening before bed. He also said that he was referring me to the local Sensory Loss Team (which I would later go on to work for) and that he wanted to complete my registration of visual impairment. This was the most painful experience for me out of everything I went through on my journey of losing my sight as I call it. I signed the certificate of visual impairment with the help of the consultant and was told that I would be registered as blind.

My world crumbled there and then and I went into shock. I couldn't wait to get out of the office, and as soon as I was out of the hospital doors I cried like a baby, and kept repeating to myself, "I'm blind, I'm blind." Thank goodness Jo was there. I found it devastating that I was now blind, as in my head blind meant you couldn't see anything, which I now know not to be true. I am also amazed that they can give you this bad news and then just show you the door. God, I like to think things have changed but from what I hear they are still doing it this way.

A few days later I received a phone call to say that the flat was ready and that we could move in the following week. I telephoned a few friends and they agreed to give me a hand. I managed to carry Jo over the threshold of the flat and then moved all the furniture in. The flat later turned out to be a nightmare: damp, noisy neighbours, and a land lord who only cared as long as he got the rent.

Weeks later my consultant examined my eyes and indicated his suspicions on a condition called Leber's Hereditary Optic Neuropathy (LHON) and told me that they wanted to do a simple blood test to confirm this. The process of elimination continued; the boxes were getting less and less.

Late one evening in December I received a phone call at home from my consultant who in his soft, kind, caring voice reported that testing of my DNA had found a fault and that it was confirmed that I had LHON and this would be confirmed by a letter in the post. I thanked him for ringing me personally and hung up. I was somewhat pleased as I now knew what was wrong with me and it felt a relief after months and months of tests. The letter came and said, "David Rosser has tested positive for the mitochondrial G➔A mutation at nucleotide 11178 which is commonly associated with Leber Hereditary Optic Neuropathy (LHON). Therefore this confirms the diagnosis of LHON in this patient."

At my next check up I was asked if I wanted genetic counseling and was told that my condition was not common and some specialists from up country would like to come and look in my eyes, to which I agreed. The specialist also asked me to go for a heart scan to ensure that there were no defects as this can be a side effect of the condition, but all was good—no defects—and they found a heart much to Jo's surprise.

The night before I had an appointment with these so called top consultants to view my optic nerve, I visited an old friend who just happened to have some marijuana. We had a good smoke that night and I went on my merry way as I had a big day in the morning. I arrived at the hospital and was shown to a large room which had a dozen or more excited consultants all queued up ready to look into my eyes. They all had total disregard for myself, not interested in who I was, they were just interested in my optic nerve and their careers. I'm not sure if they knew I had a little smoke the night before, but I'm glad I did as I think that if I wasn't so mellow that morning I probably would have told the whole lot of them what I really thought of them, which would not have been very pleasant.

I declined the genetic counseling due mainly to their arrogance; however, I agreed to a type of counseling through the hospital specializing in sight loss. The first session was a disaster as I just talked and talked and the counselor just hummed and said go on, go on, and I would have gotten more out of talking to the wall. It's not how I remember being taught counseling when I was at University. I went back the following week and started off the session by saying that it would be my last session as I felt that I did not get anything out of the first session. I picked up my coat and went and had a cup of coffee. I do hope that the woman who had done the counseling has either retired or was retrained.

Shorty afterwards I received a visit from a Rehabilitation Officer for the Visually Impaired (ROVI) and I did not like her one bit. In fact, she gave me the creeps and talked in a flat monotone voice, which was always a sign not to trust someone; it made me wonder what was she hiding. She visited me a couple more times, always in the evening and seemed to talk more about herself at times than me.

I was struggling when outdoors and had always been independent so I managed to persuade her for a mobility lesson. She felt it was too early but I felt I was more of a risk as I was always out and about and not one to sit indoors and watch life go by. The first mobility lesson was useless and we went about 20 feet to the end of my drive and back again. That just didn't whet the appetite and I was getting frustrated and despondent. How long was mobility training going to take at this rate? I would be collecting my pension before I had learned. At the next visit the ROVI never showed up; maybe the long mobility lesson had been too much for her. So after a few weeks and hearing nothing I gave her a call to find that she was unwell due to stress and I would not see her for another six months.

Thankfully a woman, Caroline, at the local job centre was very proactive and managed to get me on a work rehabilitation course with the Royal National Institute for the Blind (RNIB) at Manor House, which just so happened to be in my local town of Torquay. I was made up. Having studied Occupational Therapy and then losing my sight was a strange experience. It gave me the drive and the motivation to get back out in the world to still become an Occupational Therapist, however a visually impaired one at that, which is difficult as I trained as a sighted Occupational Therapist. The two are very different, and not only would I need to learn new skills as a newly qualified Occupational Therapist, but I would need to learn new skills as a visually-impaired person.

They fast tracked my application as Manor House was closing. It is still talked about today in the visually-impaired world as it was a Mecca for people with sight loss, leading to many relationships and people moving to Torquay following their courses there. I spent 10 weeks at Manor House, learning touch typing in 4 weeks which had previously eluded me for 3 years at University whilst I was sighted: how bizarre is that. I also learned

Information Technology (IT) skills and the use of screen reader software. I initially trained on Job Access with Speech (JAWS) before using SuperNova, which is my preference today. I also learned Braille and had mobility training which was exceptional, and counseling which was the real deal this time.

Most importantly, the best therapy was done over a cup of tea with a biscuit at break times with fellow visually-impaired students. I learned more over a cup of tea in those 10 weeks than I ever learned from any therapist or rehab worker. Now that's what I call therapy. I did however give the staff a run for their money as I remember one day being asked to put nuts on bolts to help with dexterity practice. Having trained as an Occupational Therapist I found this insulting and I didn't take this lying down because in Occupational Therapy we always used meaningful and purposeful activities. Oh the staff loved me.

Following my course I signed up at a local college to study reflexology as a stop gap to Occupational Therapy. It was a disaster and they had no idea how to meet my needs. They even tried to push me off the course, but I dug my heels in and they employed a woman who used to work at Manor House and I started to enjoy the course.

Whilst at Manor House I had applied for a grant from a charity run by Lord "S", former Photographer to the Queen, and I received a letter to say that I was successful to the tune of £2000. This enabled me to buy my laptop and the software to go with it. One of the conditions was that I had to go and meet Lord "S" at the House of Commons for lunch along with other successful candidates. "Hey, a free lunch at the House of Commons," I thought, but more importantly I could now be independent again and not have someone take my notes and research material for me. I could now do this for myself; how empowering that was.

I took my dad with me for lunch at the House of Commons and I felt a big gratitude toward Lord "S" due to what the grant had enabled me to do. This debt of gratitude soon vanished when being one of the first up to speak to him was rushed through and I overheard Lord "S" say to his entourage, "Can't you move them along faster?" like he had to be somewhere else. But the lunch was nice.

Shortly after finishing and passing the reflexology course a job came up with the local Sensory Loss Team working with visually-impaired people. I applied and got an interview in which I excelled and was offered the post of Sensory Rehabilitation worker. In the same week I learned that the love of my life Jo was pregnant and that we had an offer from the local council to move to a house, which we accepted. What a week it was turning into. We moved from the damp flat two weeks after I started my job, but all was not great in the Sensory Loss Team.

At the end of the first day I had an appointment with Jo and the mid wife and did not want to share with people yet that I was about to be a dad, so just said I had a doctor's appointment. I was on flexi-time and could leave at 4pm. I tidied my desk at the end of the day and before I knew what was happening my old rehab officer stood next to me, inches from my face, and snapped, "Where do you think you're going?" I replied that I had a doctor's appointment and was left free to go. My intuition was right the first time I had met this woman. From the frequency of her voice I knew this was not a nice woman and even though her name was not on the manager's door, she was the self-proclaimed manager. "Might is right" in her world; it was time to look for another job.

After two years of hell at this job, I received an email one day from a fellow Occupational Therapy colleague to say that a secondment within the company was coming up and I would be an ideal candidate for the job. I applied and got an interview; however, on the day of the interview I woke up with the flu. After a couple of Paracetamol I dragged myself to the interview, coughing and spluttering. I kept saying to myself I have to get this job, I have to get this job, and I answered all the questions fully and even managed to waffle which is most unlike me. But I got the job: fantastic, awesome, as the road had been so hard and long, but I had made it: I was going to be an Occupational Therapist.

On reflection I have no regrets in my life and my sight loss has changed my life profoundly. It has brought me many positive opportunities, including meeting people who I would never have met and having experiences I would never have dreamt of. My mantra of, "Better to burn up than rust away," is no more as I honour my body these days, eating a very natural diet, exercising daily as my body struggles to rid itself of toxins, and I am forced to lead a healthy lifestyle mostly.

I always knew looking back the tears would make me laugh, but I never knew looking back the laughs would make me cry, and now I live every day as if it's my last.

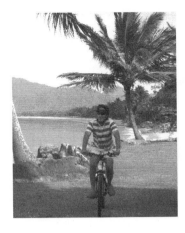
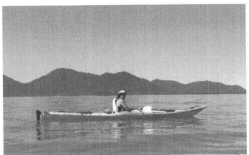

Life with **LHON**

James Crawford
Date of Birth 1964
Age of LHON onset: age 8, 1973
Mutation 11778
Place of Birth, Bethesda, Maryland, USA
Current residence, Cairns, Queensland, Australia

"Why is the teacher writing in Chinese?" I asked my friend as we sat in the back row of class on a Wednesday morning in July of 1973.

My friend laughed, "He's not."

"Yes he is," I insisted, "the first column is normal, but now he is writing Chinese."

I was sitting in the back row of a scripture class, a class I normally would never have attended. Instead, I used to go to the library every Wednesday morning. Today the library was closed, so I had to attend the scripture class. The teacher was writing on the board and we were to copy the board into our books. I recall having no problem at all with reading the first column of writing, but then half way down the second column the writing on the board became illegible and appeared to be a different language. Once the other classes began for the day, the teacher moved me to halfway down the classroom row of tables and I could see the board again. However, by afternoon, I could not read the board from halfway down the row of tables either. Only if I sat in the front row could I see the board.

I don't recall any pain or trauma before or during my vision loss. At age 8 I just thought I needed glasses, which was a horrible thought, knowing how I would be teased for wearing glasses by all the kids at school. The next day my father organized for me to see an ophthalmologist. My biggest fear was that I was going to need glasses; I really didn't want to be a "four eyes" and teased.

My mother and I were not long at the ophthalmologist as he did a few tests, looked at my eyes, and then made some phone calls before sending us upstairs to a specialist ophthalmologist. Again a few tests, a look at my eyes, a few more tests, and then the specialist tried some different lenses on me with no results. A few days later I was off to another specialist, a neurologist this time.

Obviously something was going on with me and it was more than just needing a pair of glasses. The year 1973 is a long while back, and as an 8 going on 9 year old, it's hard to recall a lot of what was going on. I remember my mother and I saw the ophthalmologist and neurologist every 2 weeks for 6 months to a year, for more tests. My father, who was a doctor, also attended many of these appointments. After the tests were done, I would always be asked to wait outside while my mother and father talked with the specialists.

The fortnightly visits to see the specialists for tests were actually not all that disturbing and even fun and rewarding in some ways. For an 8 to 9 year old it meant a day off school, and what kid doesn't want a day off school every 2 weeks? After seeing doctors we would always visit the milk bar in the foyer of the medical centre and I would have an ice cream and chocolates. Sometimes after a visit my mother and I would do fun things like go to the zoo or shopping, so I was happy to have a day off school.

I remember test after test after test. Unfortunately, in 1973 the LHON gene had not yet been discovered, so there was no genetic test to identify an LHON gene. I had numerous brain scans and brain activity graphs. Although LHON may have been considered by the specialist, with no family history

134

of vision loss and no way of diagnosing LHON for certain, doctors and my parents kept looking for an answer to why I could not see, I guess hoping we would find something that could be cured.

Every fortnight I would perform the visual field tests either on a big blackboard or on a machine that flashed dots and I had to push a button when I saw the dots. I had EEGs, PEGs, OCTs, VERs, FFAs, Angiograms, X-rays, and test after test, brain scan after brain scan. While in the hospital for the worst of all tests, I recall a group of medical students coming through and all of them looking at my eyes. I recall photographs of my eyes being taken and apparently my eyes made it into some ophthalmological journal. That was the curiosity: I could not see, but to look at my eyes even in detail, the eyes themselves appeared normal in every way.

But the worst test of all is something called a PEG. Needles were inserted into my brain and brain fluid was removed and tested. After that test I had to lie in the hospital bed and could not move a muscle without the most severe pain in my head. I am quite sure I have suffered headaches through life as a result of this test, but if not from the test, regardless I have suffered headaches since not long after losing my vision. The only treatment I received was an extended course of corticosteroids to try and prevent the vision loss from getting any worse.

I travelled with my mother and met up with my father in England for more tests in London. This included more brain scans and more sophisticated state of the art EEGs. The main purpose of the trip was to have a brain scan in the world's first CT scanner. In 1973 the CT scanner was a brand new invention and there was only one in the world. I was one of the first to be scanned and I guess I was definitely the first Australian to be scanned on a CT scanner. So we really had tried everything looking for a diagnosis. Having a father who was a doctor had meant many doors had been opened quickly and I saw the best in the world at the time.

For 25 years my condition was "Bilateral Optic Atrophy causing a loss of Central Vision from no known cause." I don't recall the vision loss starting in one eye or the other, and as I could not read the blackboard at the moment of onset, I presumed both eyes were affected at the same time. The central vision loss was worse in my right eye, though. This "Bilateral Optic Atrophy" had left me with normal peripheral vision, but almost no central vision, and a visual acuity of 2/60 in the right eye and 3/24 in the left, leaving me legally blind. Although in the first year there had been a very slight improvement in my vision, this probably can be attributed to better compensation skills by the vision I was left with.

It was not until 1998 that I got a diagnosis of LHON after an ophthalmologist made the remark on a report that "Lebers Hereditary Optic Neuropathy should be considered." The LHON gene had now been identified and there was now a test. The test was positive for LHON, and so after 25 years I finally had a diagnosis of LHON 11778. My vision has remained stable and my visual acuity and field losses today are the same as they were when I tested in 1974. So although it made no difference in the prognosis, to have a name to put to the condition and know there were others with the same condition, was a good feeling. It really did help being able to give a name to my vision loss.

I often hear people complaining about the time it takes to diagnose LHON. Well, it took 25 years for me, so people can count themselves lucky they only have to wait a few weeks or months for a positive diagnosis nowadays. Without any family history of vision loss, it is hard to identify and diagnose LHON, so it is great that there is now a way to positively identify LHON with genetic tests. Before the test was available, I'm sure hundreds of people went through life undiagnosed such as myself. I also believe doctors want to look for an alternate reason for the vision loss in case it is something that can be cured.

As I still had a touch of central vision remaining in my left eye, a big thick magnifying glass (+33) was mounted in the left side of my eyeglasses frame. However, I had no central vision at all in the right eye—there was nothing to magnify—so the right side of my glasses frame was left clear or frosted. With these glasses I could read print, but I had to be an inch away from what I was reading, my nose rubbing the book as I read. As the focus distance on the glasses is only an inch, anything further than that is blurred, so the glasses are useless for anything but reading. I could not make out any details up close without my glasses and I could not read the blackboard. I still use the same glasses today as my primary source of visual aid.

I hated so much my appearance when I had to read, I would rarely read and I didn't take the glasses out in public with me. I would always get others to read for me. It was not until my late 20s that I started carrying my glasses. For many years I would read as little as possible due to the discomfort and slowness of reading and would read only what I had to. I did not read for pleasure.

Then in 1998 while suffering deep depression, I started to read books, novels, and fiction, and although it was a strain and slow, I learnt to love reading. I got used to the strain and it no longer stops me from reading. I was never one who enjoyed audio books, as I just didn't seem to follow them and my mind would wander. But sitting and reading with my powerful glasses—with the book an inch away rubbing the end of my nose—is now one of the greatest pleasures I can think of. Once I start enjoying the book, the strain of reading seems to disappear and I can focus on the book in hand.

However, back to 1973. I can now imagine that this must have been a dreadfully worrying time for my parents and family, not knowing what was going on with their youngest of six children. All I knew was I couldn't see well anymore, I couldn't read, and that normal glasses did not help at all. But at 8 years old my biggest concern was changing schools.

I was still attending my usual local school and playing with all my local friends. However, I could no longer read the board at school, even from the front row. I recall my teacher was very nice and wanted to keep me in her class. Nonetheless, I was going blind and so I had to change to a special school.

I remember meetings with school counselors and then visiting both a School for the Blind and a school that had a Partially Sighted Unit attached to it. This I found very upsetting and disturbing as a now 9 year old. I did not want to change schools and leave all my local friends, and no way did I want to attend the Blind School with all those blind kids or the Partially Sighted Unit. I can recall so clearly seeing all these kids wearing glasses, bending over to read things, using magnifying glasses, and all of them looked like "stupid idiots." Excuse the term, but as a child in 1973, that is what I felt about the blind kids and I did not want to be part of them. To this day I still hate seeing pictures of me reading as it reminds me of all those blind kids back at that school.

The school I had to attend was a Partially Sighted Unit and was more than an hour's drive from home. So no more playing with friends before or after school, as that time was now spent travelling in cars. A driver would pick up me and a group of other partially-sighted children every morning and drive us to and from school.

Segregated schooling was the standard and accepted practice in the 1970s and I am so glad that this period of forced segregation for those with disabilities is over. My education and social abilities suffered a great deal from being forced to attend a special school and leave all my old school friends and classrooms behind.

I spent 3 years at the Partially Sighted Unit. Yes, I made friends there, but the friends were from all over the place and did not live in my local area. At the Partially Sighted Unit we did not mix with the mainstream children in the rest of the school. We had separate areas for our lunch and play, so very quickly in those school years I learnt I was different from others and shouldn't play with the mainstream kids at school. I had a nice teacher and support, but we were isolated.

Then in 1977, I was off to high school. This time it was a mainstream high school closer to where I lived, but not my local school. The high school had a Special Education teacher and a special classroom for the students with vision impairment. For the first year, math and English classes were taught by our special education teacher and we were in a special class. All our other subjects were in the mainstream school with no in-class support provided. By the third year of high school, all our classes were in the mainstream school with no support provided. Large print books, magnifying glasses, or mini-scopes were probably all that was ever provided at high school.

Being thrown into the mainstream school system after 3 years of segregation was a shock to the system. In the first week or two I tried to make friends with the mainstream students, but soon the teasing and bullying started and it was much easier to just start hanging around the vision-impaired students.

138

In class I would have to rely on a sighted friend to read the board for me or try and use my mini-scope, which is a mini telescope, but that was slow and exhausting. It was often hard to find friends who would read the board to me, because to help me meant that kid would get teased and bullied by other students for helping the partially-sighted kids.

Sports class was the worst of all. Due to having some classes with the special education teacher, my sports times were changed. So rather than doing sports with my homeroom class, I had to join another sports class, and that class had all the tough kids in it. Every sports session I would be bullied, stirred, and isolated by the tough kids. I was always the last to be picked for a team and laughed at when I couldn't see a ball or do something correctly. I hated sports as a result, and after getting an ankle injury at home, I managed to avoid sports for the next year. I don't recall enjoying much of high school, and in 1981 I left school.

What I had wanted to do after leaving school was to work on boats, to be a shipwright. My mother assisted me, and while I was still in school, we went all over the place visiting boatyards and applying or asking for an apprenticeship, but with no success at all. Eventually I got a job as a screen printer's assistant and left school. I had not actually told the employer that I had a vision problem when applying and getting the job. That job only lasted a few weeks as I found the vision challenges too difficult to perform my job properly. My employer was sympathetic and offered to keep me on and assist me, but I was a mess inside my head and just had to get out.

So I was 17: no job, no school. I really didn't know what to do, as I knew my head space was not good, but I was not willing to tell anyone that I was not coping. I had to be tough. So the next 8 or so years I went on with trying this and that, taking courses, jobs, changing my mind, playing in bands, and working with bands. The only thing I really liked doing and which kept me stable was sailing and ocean yacht racing.

In the 1980s, I played in bands as a drummer, then a singer, and then just started hanging around and working sometimes with bands. I earned an Audio Engineering Certificate, thinking with my vision I could work with sound, but the music industry was not for me. I took a year of Naval Architecture, but prior to computers the line drawings required were far too difficult for me to do with accuracy, so another idea for a career was left behind.

I worked as a Clerk in the Public Service, but I knew that job was not for me. I also felt disheartened when three other clerks who had started with me had all moved up the ranks while I was still doing the same job. Prior to computers a lot of office work was very difficult for me. I left the public service job and went back to school to get my university entrance. I didn't know what I wanted to do, but I thought that if I studied I may work it out.

I found the education system again very hard and did not do well the first year. The second year I just focused on three subjects for university entrance and did OK. I do recall the frustration I used to go through during classes, using my mini-scope to read the board and then write in my books. It was so hard, I really don't think anyone ever realises that using a mini-scope and then putting powerful glasses on and writing is as hard as it is. The strain on my eyes and me mentally was immense. I recall so many classes where I just wanted to run from the classroom as the stress was just so incredibly high trying to read and write.

I had thought I might study Earth Sciences and Coastal Geomorphology or Meteorology, but the idea of trying to keep up with the entire math and reading lecture screens was too much to bear. So I didn't go to University at that stage and study something of interest to me. The idea of studying at University just seemed too stressful prior to the availability of modern technology. And as it turns out, a lot of my life has been involved in the environmental movement and stopping coastal developments, so a degree in Earth Sciences would have been excellent, "but them's the breaks."

So for most of the 1980s I was pretty much wandering from this to that, trying to find myself and what I could do in life with a vision loss. However, I sailed every chance I got. I ocean raced, I cruised, worked around boats and in a few boat yards. I spent a lot of time restoring an old 1920s Gaff Rigger, the family boat, and then sold that and bought a 26-foot yacht of my own. I sailed that yacht of mine a lot and did so much work to it. I did have plans of just heading off sailing to see where it would take me. I studied my Master V Mariners course for the knowledge it provided, but I knew I could not get the Masters license due to my vision impairment.

However, at 16 I managed to get my Power Boat Drivers License. I had studied for the test and knew I would pass the theory without a problem, but I also knew I would fail the eye sight test. On the day of my test I went armed with a letter from my doctor stating he considered my vision impairment good enough to allow me to drive a small power boat. The examiner on the day also had watched me grow up on the waterfront and knew I was a good boat handler, and he agreed to give me a license, but warned me not to drive too fast. In all the years of having that license I have had only one accident back in 1989 and I was not at fault. I feel I know my limitations in a power boat and pretty much have stuck to them.

The year 1988 was a year of great excitement, learning and challenges. It started with some wonderful work on a 30 metre luxury motor yacht, the Antipodean, as a deckhand. I thought, "Hey, this is it, it's finally happening. If I can stay on this boat I can make a life out of it." Very sadly, that was not to be the case.

A local skipper had been hired by the owners to work with the boat's main skipper. This local skipper had taught me for a few weeks at navigation school, and his opinion was that I should not be in the course, that I should not be on the water. When he came on board the Antipodean, he made sure I was fired soon after. Of course the excuse of not needing the extra crew was used; however, I knew what the real reason was. There are people who give you a go and realise you are capable, and then there are others, who without knowing you or your skills, write you off as blind and therefore useless. Definitely a blind person does not belong on a boat, according to some skippers.

I didn't know what 1988 was going to have in store for me now. Then I got a position as crew on a 44 foot racing yacht my neighbour skippered. My neighbour Jamie was a year or two younger than me, but he knew me well and knew I was good crew. We sailed off for a 400 mile ocean race up the coast, and we came in third and were all pleased. The winds were from the south and none of us felt like going home, so we just kept racing. Eventually we raced all the way to Papua New Guinea and returned to Sydney, winning many of the races we entered. It was a great sail and taught me a great deal, but it also taught me that my vision was going to be a major problem once I got out of the local waters I knew so well.

In the years 1988 and 1989 I did not know what I wanted to do other than sailing. I did it all the time and spent much of my time working on and maintaining my boat. I sailed across the Coral Sea to Vanuatu as crew on a 57-foot yacht and it made me realise how difficult my dream of sailing my own yacht to new ports was going to be. The sailing in the open ocean and storms and calms did not bother me: it was wonderful out there with water in all directions. Hand steering a yacht in all conditions and keeping on a good compass course was wonderful and once I had the feel of the boat and the boat in trim, I could keep a good true course without watching the compass. Being able to see the compass was difficult, having to get an inch away from it, but I managed. The difficulty I had was entering new ports and following navigation marks. This was all before GPS and affordable radars and sonar's and so much modern equipment.

Most of the time my vision impairment was not an issue or even considered: I was just part of the crew. By sailing, week in and week out, I soon gained experience and learnt a great deal. Regularly I would be given the responsibility of taking the yacht from the mooring to the club, and although vision impaired, I also was given responsibility for my neighbour's yachts and never put a scratch on one of them.

I raced and sailed both in Sydney and in Pittwater north of Sydney. At 3:00 in the morning, in 40 kts and 7 metre waves, being up the bow and changing a headsail, holding on as the boat would go under waves and then working furiously before the next wave, there was no thought of being vision impaired. I just did the sail change, hung on, and worked just the same as any fully sighted crew member. I raced in some very competitive classes, such as Etchells, with skippers who gave me a chance and did not discriminate.

Sure I could not see too well, but with a pair of binoculars and keeping a good watch I managed to sail all over Sydney Harbour even on weekends with all the boat traffic around. Binoculars were my vision aid, and although I could not see the details of other boats, I could see them and avoid them when needed. And when out in the open ocean and under sail, there was a lot less to hit and I could focus on sailing and the feel of the boat.

As I said before, I was lucky enough to ocean race all the way from Sydney to Papua New Guinea and return. It was a great voyage and I learnt so much and honed my sailing skills. I now felt confident in any sailing condition and could navigate with assistance. A crew member who was trying to put me down said a blind man should not be on a yacht. However, he had the tables turned on him when I adopted the name "Blindman" for the next 3 months of racing and demonstrated my skills were equal to those with vision time and time again, particularly at night. At night a sailor must use his peripheral vision as much as possible. At night the boat is dark and so is the environment and by utilising peripheral vision a sailor can spot unlit obstacles far better than trying to stare at them using central vision. So at night I sometimes even had an advantage. It took the crew and skipper a while to trust that I could see unlit objects before they often did.

On the open ocean my vision was no issue at all and I loved being out there, but my mental health was in turmoil. While I did not talk of my mental health issues, I started to take control of my vision impairment medical history and got all my records and read through them all. As I had only been 8 at the time of onset, I had never known all the details of what went on. To read all these records was a very good but disturbing experience. For the first time in 17 years of being vision impaired, I recall being away on my boat alone, reading the records, and crying, feeling so depressed. I had always been someone who either had control of or acted as though I had control of my vision impairment and coped with it well, not letting it stop me, but suddenly that all seemed to change. For the first time I felt blind and that my disability had control of me rather than me controlling my disability.

I sold my yacht in 1994 and have not owned a yacht since. I have not sailed much in the last 15 years, but do get out from 6 to 10 times a year for a sail out to the reef on my neighbour's Catamaran and some fun snorkelling. Sure I do not see the coral and fish the way others do, but I still see enough to appreciate their beauty and enjoy swimming around in unspoiled reefs. I've done a bit of racing with the Cairns Yacht Club, but cruising is more my style nowadays.

When I started sailing in the 1970s there was no sailing for the blind or disabled, so I always sailed and competed with fully sighted people. I never really did any other sport. Ball games were out and competing against sighted peers never seemed really fair or equal. But in sailing, I could hold my own against many sighted sailors. Close quarter navigation and following a compass course or finding a mark or buoy were difficult. But once I get the feel of the boat, holding a course is easy and does not require a constant check on the compass. As yacht racing is mostly a crewed sport, I was part of a crew, so any short comings my vision caused could be compensated for by a sighted crew member.

Nowadays blind sailing and disabled sailing exist; however, I have not gotten involved. If I lived in Sydney, maybe I would engage in some of the blind and disabled sailing teams. Regardless, I've never been good at being part of a vision impaired or disabled group. I have never really felt I fit in with these groups because I can walk around and do not look impaired and I have learnt how to compensate so well with vision impairment, I don't feel I belong. I also find whenever I am with other people with disabilities, I am more aware of my disability and I guess I don't like being aware that I have a disability.

To keep hearing, "You can do whatever you want to do," used to and still does annoy me at times. It's almost more of a throw away phrase than reality. Yes, one can do anything they want, but if you are vision impaired there are things that cannot be done: driving, for instance, or being the commercial master of a vessel or an aircraft pilot. Sure there are ways around things, challenges that can be met, modifications, and special equipment, but that all adds a great deal to the stress of doing just about anything at all. I believe if you have a passion for something, you are far more likely to succeed in that area, but succeeding may require changes to the way you do things, and doing it differently from sighted people.

I have found life being vision impaired very stressful. For many years I would not have admitted it or even realised the level of tension it caused. As I lost my central vision at age 8, being vision impaired was pretty much all the life I knew. I just kept doing things, but regardless, all activities were and are more difficult with vision impairment. From the age of 8 until 30 I did not seek help to deal with the stress and depression that a vision-impaired life created. I knew I was stressed, but I was not ready to admit it or acknowledge the depression for many years. At the age of 25, I really knew my mental health was suffering and that my adult life being vision impaired was not going to be as easy as it was being a teenager and adolescent. So many things

I wanted to do just seemed so difficult to achieve, and I wanted to succeed, but I knew my emotional energy just didn't have the strength.

In 1990, feeling totally lost, I was encouraged by family to enroll in University for a Diploma of Teaching Early Childhood. I had always enjoyed spending time with my young nieces and nephews and it seemed like a fair degree to obtain. I knew teaching was not for me, but without any other ideas, I persisted and completed my degree in Early Childhood Education and eventually began work as an early childhood teacher in the day care setting.

University stressed me terribly. I found trying to do all the work at the same pace as other students so draining. Everything I did would take longer, and although my outcome was the same as for the sighted students, it took me a lot more effort for the same result. It was tiring.

At least in the second year of University laptop computers were now available. The Government, through the Commonwealth Rehabilitation Service, bought me a laptop and special software. With a laptop, taking notes and writing became so much easier than the old fashioned way of tape recording lectures and going home to type them up. The laptop made such a difference. It's hard to imagine, but I was the only student at our University campus with a laptop, as they were so rare in 1991.

University was difficult but well worth doing. I was given very little support by any University disability officers. I managed with my monocular, tape recorder, laptop and a great deal of assistance from my mother with her reading books onto tape and assisting with course work.

The Government helped by buying the laptop for me, providing financial assistance to study, and paying for books. I would get extra time for exams and the option to type rather than write on the exam papers.

After 3 years of very hard work I had a degree in Early Childhood Education. Straight out of University I gained employment at one of the best day care centres in the country and not far from home. It was a maternity leave contract for 12 months or more. I had done two practicum at the centre and they knew me well, and after the job interview I was told I had secured the position. But then everything was thrown into the air by discrimination.

During a phone inquiry about my position, a personnel officer from the Council that operated the day care centre made a big error and said, "We can't employ a teacher who is blind." So, there came the reality of working as a teacher. I had my degree, but I still had to prove I was capable in quite a different manner than my fully-sighted colleagues; so much for Equal Employment Opportunity. In fact, a few years later when trying to get work in the public school system, again I had to go through a whole series of interviews and medicals to ascertain my ability to work as a teacher.

I certainly stood up for my rights, but there was difficulty. Although by 1994 the Federal and State governments had Equal Employment Opportunity laws, the Council I was to work for was not yet adopting the policies. This situation of the Council being outside of Federal and State laws was to be changing soon and the Council recognised their obligation to employ me. After several months and discussion with the Human Rights and Equal Opportunity Commission, I was employed as the teacher for the 4-year-old group.

However, it was still not truly equal. Part of my contract required me to report weekly to the Director with progress reports and need for assistance. This was not such a bad thing. It is good to have meetings with superiors to make sure you are getting the assistance you may require, but it was the manner in which it was done at the time that was not equal as compared to fully sighted employees. All first year teachers should be subjected to that style of supervision.

So I worked for a year in that centre with the 4 year olds and in the 1-year-old room. Sometimes I liked it and felt that my training was paying off. I had my degree and now a job. But another part of me found it so very difficult. Being responsible for the safety and well being of twenty-five 4 year olds, even with assistants, was still very stressful. I had to find strategies to record and monitor all the little things a teacher has to do. I had a tape recorder in my pocket for notes and I walked around constantly so I could supervise the children. Even explaining my vision loss to the children, their parents, and to other staff was stressful. I never minded explaining, but if I was not vision impaired I would not have to do this. So suddenly, on top of my job, I am also having to describe my disability and having to always find strategies and ways to do things in order to succeed over the challenges life has brought me.

In 1994 I moved from Sydney to the tropics of northern Australia. Here was a whole new world to find myself lost in. I had wanted to live in the Cairns area for many years and had considered the way my vision impairment would affect moving and living independently. Due to my concerns I had made plans for the move with friends and was planning at least a 3-month adjustment period, where the friends would be there to help.

I moved to a small coastal town, but then the friends who had done all the planning and moved north with me stayed only 3 days and then left with no explanation, leaving me alone in a remote town 3,000 km from home. I had wanted to move to the tropics, but I had not planned on doing it all suddenly on my own.

I had a push bike and the local store was not far to ride or walk to, so shopping was not too hard, but the local store was limited and trips to bigger towns were needed. Without a car and no public transportation, this was mighty hard. I met nice people who did help out and would take me with them on their shopping trips, but not being able to drive myself, I was not independent.

I also discovered how although I was a great boat handler and could navigate well in Sydney and surrounding waters, once I was in this new part of the world it was much harder. I still managed and used to take my small boat out to different islands all on my own or take my sea kayak for paddles along the Mangrove-lined coast.

Depression was becoming a major problem for me and I now sought help, but in a remote town, help was limited. There were many personal factors to the depression, not related to LHON, but also it was awareness that all my dreams and desires for life were not falling into place and one big reason was being vision impaired. I had spent 20 years finding ways around problems and finding different ways to do things, I had accepted the challenges of being vision impaired and not let them beat me.

I often used to say to people that being vision impaired did have its problems and when a wall was thrown in my path I would just climb the wall, walk around the wall, or find a door in that wall and beat the challenge. I had succeeded in many areas like sailing and gaining a university degree, but I was also tired and worn out from continually having to find the alternate ways to do things and having to ask others to help. I had coped with being vision impaired for so long that it was also almost impossible to start telling people I was no longer coping with being vision impaired. It was far easier to talk about issues that others understood like relationship problems and general life issues than it was to talk about "hating" being blind.

As my depression deepened and mania started to creep in, one morning I got involved in being an environmentalist. A knock on the door one day, when I was truly at my utter lowest and could see no reason to keep living, brought a big change in life again.

I then got involved in action to protect the environment of Hinchinbrook Island and surrounds, the Dugongs, and wildlife that call the area home. This area was almost pristine and an area I had loved for many years, and a huge marina resort development threatened this unique natural environment. I had video cameras, mobile phones, and boats, all of which were useful to the campaign and I got involved. A few days later saw me and a few others standing in front of bulldozers and excavators attempting to stop the clearing of a Mangrove forest.

Here being vision impaired did not bother me. I would walk right up to a machine and just stand there or move to block its path. Being vision impaired also had its drawbacks as I did not see unfriendly workers coming toward me until it was too late and then I would cop a lot of verbal abuse and minor assaults. Here, I was part of a small group leading a major environmental campaign and I was legally blind and it didn't matter at all that I was vision impaired. With a group, I just did what had to be done.

I soon knew I could not stay in the remote town and moved on to Cairns. I returned to teaching and would travel by taxi to and from work each day. Again I felt the stress of teaching and the difficulties of not being able to see the children well. This added a great deal of strain to what was often an enjoyable job. Sure the children all got used to the way I read and how I would read the words then show the pictures to them. But I still felt so unlike other teachers: I had to do things differently and that made me different. I did not want to be different.

Again, depression took its hold on me after teaching for a couple of years and, combined with other personal and vision issues, I stopped teaching. And since that time in 1998, depression has been my major disability, not the vision impairment. Due to major depression I returned to Sydney and family for help. There were other factors to the depression than being vision impaired, but it was a contributing factor. Treatment in Sydney eventually led to Electro Convulsive Therapy and I started to lift out of the blackest depression.

Returning to Cairns a few years later I started working in an office, and although I could do everything required, I was slower than a sighted person would be and this really annoyed me. Once again so much more effort and time were required for me to obtain the same level as a sighted person.

Once a bit healthier, I returned to teaching but this time as a Special Education teacher working with students with intellectual impairments, vision impairments, and speech language impairments. Again I found teaching so stressful, just monitoring and working with students was hard. If they had a question and wanted me to look at what they had written, it was difficult: out came the glasses, and I read what they had written back to them. Other teachers, though, could just sit with a student and read the writing, show the student where they had gone wrong and correct them. For me it was a whole series of steps to read the students' work, and then help them correct it.

Working with vision impaired students sounded like a great idea; however, it was particularly hard as both students and I could not see things. It stressed me and was not good for my mental health. In 2004 I stopped teaching and have never returned to it.

Maybe if I had a passion for teaching I would have coped with it, and found more ways to deal with all the challenges being vision impaired threw my way, but I did not have a passion for teaching and the best thing I could do was stop teaching. It took several years to get rid of the letdown I felt in myself for no longer teaching. I had to remind myself that teaching was not the right job for me regardless of vision impairment. Even if I could see I would not have wanted to remain a teacher.

Can a blind man coordinate an Art Exhibition? Of course he can and that was my life for 2005. I had never done anything like it before, but the call went out for someone to coordinate the Dugongs of Hinchinbrook 2 Exhibition and I accepted the challenge. There were often laughs about a blind man running the art show, but why not? And indeed I worked closely with a small group of people to have the most successful art exhibition Cairns had ever seen and also the most successful art show fundraiser imaginable, with sales totalling over $100,000. I was on a high through all of this and being vision impaired didn't matter. I was part of a team that worked hard and was successful.

I needed a job though, and from 2004 to 2005 I applied for over 50 jobs and didn't make it to the interview stage on a single one. This was depressing and I realised I had to just start my own business. For the last 6 years I have owned and operated on my own a dog boarding and walking business. I have also branched into holiday property management in the last couple of years. I live alone in my own house and live independently. I do my own entire cooking, cleaning, washing, gardening, etc. I now do my grocery shopping on-line so that has taken away one major stress.

Shopping with vision impairment is a problem. To go to a supermarket and try and find items is not much fun at all. I have shopped at the same two stores for many years, so I have learnt the layouts, but if there is something that I don't usually buy, finding it is difficult. Either I search by looking close at the shelves, bending down or stretching up, or I ask for help. But to see or compare prices, or to notice that something is on special, or to just be tantalized by the sight of something you would not normally buy, just is not part of the shopping experience. For much of the last 16 years I have shopped on my own and found all that I need, but not necessarily what I want.

Transport to and from the shops has also always been a bit of a problem. I use taxis, but sometimes the wait for a taxi to get home from the shopping centre could be up to 40 minutes and that is more than annoying. For me it always made me feel blind. For a while I shopped with a friend and that made it easier, but not independent.

Recently I have changed all that shopping experience stress into something far more civilised. Internet on-line supermarket shopping and home delivery have made such a world of difference to me. To be able to go on-line and shop for groceries has been a truly liberating experience. I now feel free to find what I want easily, to see specials, to compare prices, to browse the items, and to impulse buy food items I had not thought of. To shop on-line, my experience is the same as the experience of a sighted shopper, so I truly feel equal and enjoy the experience.

There is no doubt at all that technology in the last 20 years has made a world of difference to those with vision impairments. In the 1970s and 1980s only talking books and magnifying glasses existed. With the 1990s came technology and what a difference it has made to so many people.

When I first got a laptop in 1990, I had a screen reader and large print programs that were so primitive compared to today. A very useful and necessary skill has been the ability to touch type. I was taught touch typing and Braille in the early years of losing my vision. The Braille has never been of use to me, but learning to touch type is invaluable. These days I use my powerful glasses and sit an inch away from the screen. I have a gas lift monitor arm that brings the screen out to me so I do not have to bend to it. For many years I would struggle and bend over to read the screen and cause great strain to my back and neck, but discovering the gas lift monitor arm was just wonderful and has made using the computer so much easier.

I figure the simpler the technology I use the less things there are to go wrong. It also means I can use other computers that do not have special software on them. For many years I thought there was no way I could read a computer screen with my glasses and the strain of sitting an inch from the screen would be too much to cope with. But I discovered that I found it easier to use my glasses and more efficient to navigate around the computer than it was to use special screen readers, etc.

I am sure I would benefit from getting some of the new technology and it would make my life easier and maybe soon I will. The technology I look forward to getting is the technology that is now available for yachts which would allow me to navigate and sail while being vision impaired. These include talking compasses, GPSs, HD radar and sonar, mini-cameras and large monitor displays. Although I sailed without these new technologies, they sure would make life easier and hopefully give me sailing independence.

We often hear about people with disabilities who achieve greatness and do amazing things despite their impairments. Yet having a disability is exactly that, a disability. Someone with impairment should not always have to be succeeding in something or be strong. It's also about living with the disability. Whether disabled or not, some people will do amazing things, whereas others will just live their lives day to day. Someone who is coping with a disability should be praised and used as a role model as well. At the same time, those not coping should receive understanding.

I often think having LHON as my vision impairment is harder because I do not look or act blind, as I walk without a cane and I appear sighted unless I need to read something. I do not attract the attention and assistance of others without having to first explain, "I am vision impaired. Can you help?"

Although LHON is a hereditary condition passed down the maternal mitochondrial line, the hereditary part has never seemed to be an issue in my family. Maybe because for 25 years without a positive diagnosis, the hereditary part was irrelevant as no one else in the family had ever had vision problems. Looking back along the maternal line there is no history of vision impairment, and I have three brothers and a sister, and my sister has a son and daughter. I am the only one in the family to have developed a vision loss and yet all the maternal family apparently carry the mitochondrial mutation.

However, none of my family has ever shown much concern over this hereditary fact. I am glad they consider LHON in this way. In a family where there has been only one case of vision loss, it seems to me such a waste of energy to worry about LHON when there is so much else to worry about in life.

We now know of some things to avoid as they may be possible triggers to developing LHON. We hear the phrase "avoid environmental toxins," such as all types of smoke. Of course we should not smoke, and yet we continue to live in cities with high pollution and high environmental toxins in the everyday air we breathe. There seems to be no conclusive answer as to what sets off LHON, and the list of possible triggers just keeps getting longer. Yet to live life in the modern world, we are exposed to so many environmental toxins in everyday living; it just seems that living a good healthy, happy life is one of the best things that can be done. Stress is also listed as a possible trigger, and if we are stressed about what may be causing LHON, then that in itself seems to be a possible trigger.

Overall, coming up on 39 years of being vision impaired because of LHON, life is what it is. I do not like having vision impairment. I cannot imagine anyone liking having a disability, but I do accept it, because apart from the first 8 years, my life has been a life of vision impairment. So I do not know a different type of life. I cannot compare my life to someone else's, disabled or non-disabled. My life being vision impaired is my life and the only one who has lived it is me. I have had up times and down times, I've had VERY UP times and VERY DOWN times, an ocean of a life with storms and calms, just like anyone else has.

I am glad I live in a developed country and that services have been available to me over the years. Whether it is from the organisations set up to assist the vision impaired, such as the Royal Blind Society or Vision Australia, or from the government in the form of Social Security, all assistance has helped me to live my life. In Australia I receive a pension, half price taxis, free or subsidised medical treatment, prescription medicine subsidized, and free travel on all forms of public transport. All these things do not make up for being vision impaired, but they do help live a better life as a person with vision impairment. But above all the governmental and non-governmental help, the biggest support would have to be my brothers and sister, my father for providing so well for us, and my mother who has always helped me in every part of life.

I have never called myself or considered myself blind. I use the term legally blind. But as a rule I used the term partially sighted in the early days and now vision impaired. As I can walk around without bumping into things and people who don't know me would not know I am vision impaired unless they see me read something, it's always seemed more appropriate to say vision impaired, not blind. If you tell someone you're blind, their immediate image is of someone with no vision at all, and for most LHON affected people that is not the case. Peripheral vision remains so I have always preferred vision impaired.

I have good peripheral vision and see objects without being able to identify them, but I can walk and ride a push bike without bumping into things. I have no central vision in the right eye, but a touch in the left, and with both eyes open I cannot see details, but I can see well enough to get around. In the left eye, with a touch of central vision, things are blurry but with no details, but something is there. With the right eye, there is no central vision, so there is nothing at all in the centre: not black, not white, just nothing.

Over the years I have looked into many alternate therapies hoping for a cure, such as chiropractors, acupuncture, naturopathy, homeopathy, vitamin therapies, spiritual healing, Reiki, eye exercises, etc. Nothing has ever made any difference to my vision. I have had my phases of looking into anything that may provide a cure and my phases of accepting that my eyesight is the way it is.

We now live in very exciting times, with knowledge of the mitochondria and some of its functions. Gene therapies and drugs are being developed that may soon stop LHON from developing and may provide some improvement and I believe will soon provide a cure for LHON. The knowledge on LHON seems to have snowballed in the last few years and so much is now known and each day seems to bring new understandings of LHON.

If I could be cured tomorrow I would not hesitate and would enjoy being able to see. However, I also manage life the way I see it now. I have done some amazing things, like solo sailing and ocean racing with great crews in great races, and in good weather and bad. I have played in bands, worked on boats, stood in front of bulldozers as an environmentalist, gained a degree from University, and worked as a teacher in early childhood and high school special education. Nowadays I run my own dog boarding and holiday property management businesses and survive.

I own my own house in a good beach side suburb in the tropics of northern Australia and manage all my day-to-day activities independently. I cook, bake and clean for myself, wash and tidy without help, garden, mow the lawn and do the lawn edging with an electric trimmer. I cannot see the end of the trimmer properly, but I can hear when I am hitting concrete or grass and with practice I learnt to use the equipment and cut a straight edge by ear, not sight. I use a computer, I build simple websites, and I keep busy. I have a few friends who help with transport when needed or for special shopping trips, and life with LHON goes on day after day.

So have I met the challenges of being vision impaired? Definitely YES, I certainly have. Life is not the way I planned or imagined it would be, but that goes for people regardless of a vision loss or not. The life I currently have is OK and I meet and beat almost all the challenges the day throws my way.

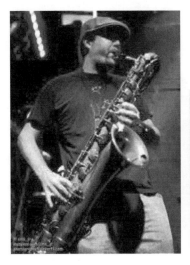
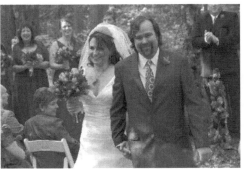

Before the Explosion (1999)

"I remember when, gazing at the sky
I would sit and wonder, 'What's out there for me?'
How could I have known that in just a day
I'd no longer have my precious sight?
Never drive again. Where are all your friends?
This is who you are now, so get used to it.
Now I waste my days staring at the sky
But that's all I need now isn't that right?

Yeah right!

These days can't last forever, or so they say.
Only the Winter can turn to Spring one day.

There are two paths that my future leads me towards.
Anything is better than I'm seeing now.
And if nothing ever really changes for me,
We all die someday, someday . . ."

    -Larry Byrne, "Turbulent Vision", c. 2002

It was a typically beautiful July day in 1999 which found us travelling in Nags Head, North Carolina. Six members of the band Jepetto, en route to a gig at The Pit, riding in the giant aquamarine vehicle we affectionately called "Falcor." Falcor is named after the flying dog in the movie "The Never Ending Story." I was doing the driving as usual, excited for the adventures we were sure to have in the new van.

I had purchased the van just days before, a solution to the impracticalities of taking a musical act on the road in a convoy of small vehicles. Now all the equipment and players could ride together and share one gas bill.

My brother says I could have been a truck driver. I drove *everywhere*. It was not uncommon for me to pick up and drive to Philadelphia or West Virginia just for fun! I could make a thirteen hour drive with one stop and still drive more when I got there. I always found it very soothing to unite with the machine and embark on a new journey. I had good music to listen to in a climate controlled chariot, and all the freedom a man could desire.

On the side of the road in Nags Head there is a narrow shoulder. It is not a paved beach town where sidewalks run the entire length. The shoulder is busy with vacationers lugging beach chairs and umbrellas, drawn to the wonderful wide beaches and pleasant ocean surf.

It was dusk, the day was still hot, and the beachgoers were returning to their cars and hotels along the highway. Without the burst of air that hit them suddenly, the pedestrians would not have known how close the careening van came to striking them as they hauled their bags home from the sandy beach.

Inside the van a commotion ensued . . .

"Whoa!"

"That was close!"

"Hey, you almost hit those people!"

My response, "What people?"

That was the last time I drove a car. My days of gallivanting around the country were over at the tender age of 18. I would never again pick up my friends after work, I would never again drive out to Interstate 81, the mountain highway, just to see the autumn trees. I was exiled to my parent's house, "up the proverbial estuary without a means of locomotion." Being accustomed to immense independence, this was a tough pill to swallow.

The first sign of something wrong with my vision occurred in the cold early months of 1999. I had a full time job working at Windermere Information Technology Systems in Annapolis. It was a terrific job! Writing and testing software for really advanced hardware was part of my daily life. The most notable program I wrote was a remote control suite for units which can decipher encoded digital information on analog waveforms. It was very stimulating, but when the large contract I was working on ended I was laid off.

I really was not a stellar employee, so no grudge remains on my part. I was often late to work and took long lunches. I was only 18 years old; my work ethic had not matured. I had dropped out of the University of Maryland after one year in the Electrical Engineering program. For someone who graduated high school a year early with 30 college credits, I was sure taking my time getting acquainted with the world, but it was fun. The loss of my day job enabled me to pursue music whole-heartedly.

Sometimes when sitting at my desk at Windermere, the text on the computer screen would appear to glow. A yellowish glow was noticeable in my right eye. I thought it was a combined side effect of not sleeping enough and staring at a computer screen eight hours a day. I began to notice when driving that if I closed one eye and then the other the lines on the road had that same yellow-purple glow especially at night.

After returning from Nags Head, the next important journeys of my life would begin with my first visit to an eye doctor. I had always had perfect 20/20 vision and a photographic memory. I was the type of person who would recognize a stranger having seen them only once before. It wouldn't be long before my closest friends were unrecognizable to me, and casual acquaintances were calling me rude for not saying hello to them.

Luckily, Doctor Rosenberg was able to give a preliminary diagnosis of Leber's Heredity Optical Neuropathy (LHON) disease the very same day. Of course further testing was required to be sure, but his familiarity helped steer us in the right direction at the very first sign of a problem. I would later learn that my genetic marker for LHON is at nucleotide position 14484.

In the recent past, medical science was unfamiliar with mitochondrial disease, and symptoms like mine would typically evoke a diagnosis of multiple sclerosis (MS). My mother told me for the first time about a great uncle George who had lost his vision, and been diagnosed as having MS. We began to realize that his was a misdiagnosis, later confirmed by DNA testing which revealed the family wide mutation which was wreaking havoc on my sight.

In the coming years I would spend a lot of time in the car with my mother. We drove to Doctor Shalom Kellman who is a neuro-ophthalmologist. Dr. Kellman was more familiar with Leber's disease and had other patients with the same disease. During the decline of my eyesight he recorded the lapsing visual fields, and watched my optic nerves die with that intensely bright bar of light. Dr. Kellman could offer no reassurance of any hope or treatment, although he was a kind and knowledgeable man. He clinically recorded the demise of the person I had once been.

The next trip we went on would be to see the experts in the field. Like the boating vacations of my youth, this time it would be both of my parents driving me. We drove all the way to Boston to see Dr. (???) at (???), there were so many doctor visits. This is about the time I really started to disassociate with the disease. At first I was able to cope with the stark finality of the diagnosis. It was just some event that happened, and this was how it would be forever more. The state sent in some vocational and life rehabilitation counselors who were all very sweet, caring people.

For the first time in my life I began to meet a lot of blind people, and I always admired their ability to face life, and overcome their impairment. I tried all the colored cellophanes which supposedly increase contrast for reading. I learned to read Braille, although I never used it to read any books. The only time it came in handy was when my niece was role-playing Helen Keller and I wrote her classmates names on a 3x5 card in Braille for her to hand out. At least the second grade class enjoyed my Braille training.

One counselor who came to visit me at home had a great solution to help me. After losing my sight I began to burn myself often while pouring boiling water into teacups, or my French press coffee maker. Being unable to see when the container was full, I would overfill it and freshly boiled water would cover my hand and arm. She taught me to measure the water to be boiled using the container that would ultimately hold it, thus ensuring there was never an excess of water with which to burn myself. I will always remember this lesson (although I forget her name). It is wonderful that there are people who give their time helping people adjust to dramatic changes like this.

A vocational counselor introduced me to the Job Access with Speech (JAWS) screen reading software. At the time there was no embedded feature in the operating system to read out loud what appears on the screen, or to echo what letters and words you type. My father bought an IBM PC jr way back in 1982, so I had been using computers for as long as I can remember. The graphic technology was really coming to a great place and I had been doing graphic design to support my musical projects for a long time. I did a lot of programming for fun, modifying the code of games I would play, and things like that.

If you've ever tried to write a computer program on a screen reader, you know it is no easy task. The abbreviations and identifiers used in typical programming languages confuse a screen reader, so I had to give up on that. The graphic design came to a halt for obvious reasons. During these years I used the computer mainly to browse the Internet; the screen reader did a fantastic job with web pages. I spent my days learning about great pianists from the jazz and classical idioms. I also used JAWS to write a lot of poetry, all too morose and frantic to share. I can still hear that creepy computer voice reading back those hopeless stanzas; it made it seem all the more desperate.

There was a theory that a B12 deficiency could contribute to vision loss. There were no medical studies to show that B12 shots would have any impact, but I wanted to try something to help my body fight the vision loss. So there I was giving myself B12 shots into the hip hoping this would somehow alter the course of the Leber's disease, but it had no effect whatsoever.

I thought I was doing pretty well adapting, but there were cracks developing in my foundation. Certain agonies of losing your sight cannot be dissolved simply with a positive attitude. I tried to be the best person I could be. More accurately, I tried to be the same person I always had been, and it was not working.

May God and my family forgive me: one day I decided to swallow a bottle of pills. I don't even know what I hoped would happen at that point. Anything seemed like it would be better than the life I was living. Luckily I told my friend Chris Hartman, who had stopped by to play some music, and he told my parents. My next trip was in a different kind of van.

Time really stands still when you are riding in an ambulance. Your mind swirls with thoughts of how stupidly you have acted, how weak of a person you are, what a disappointment you are, and every regret your memory can render. Funny thing is it was not even my darkest day, it was just a punctuation to a period filled with miserable days.

I cannot imagine how painful it must have been for my mother. Her father had killed himself and I think I romanticized it a little bit. I can never apologize for what I did that day; there is no reckoning that can account for it. I will never forgive myself.

They prescribed me those weird anti-depression pills to which I was no stranger. I stopped taking them like I always did. I would rather feel pain than feel nothing at all. I gave up on everything I cared for, I turned away my friends. I turned away my family, I started to drink a lot. I quit Jepetto on August 2nd 2001, my 21st birthday. I left them with Falcor to continue on their way with the Warped Tour, and I headed home on the train, in bitter defeat from Pittsburgh.

Au bord de l'eau (At the Water's Edge)

Walking like the nomad of antiquity, the dumbfounded wanderer, the gypsy, the saunterer will take you to places not mentioned on any map. The sidewalks stretch for miles, a neglected wasteland where none you know tread regularly. The government mandates that these concrete arteries be laid ad nauseam for the benefit of those who have no choice but to traverse them.

Walking the grim gauntlet, an overwhelming paradox unfolds before you. The beauty of the world is inescapable, it reaches out and tickles your ankles as you brush "past the pit where the asphalt flowers grow" in their spacious square centimeters. The spirits move the air around you, sometimes to a frenzy which can send the bravest soul wincing against their fury. The sky is endless, and sometimes mocks the most beautiful paintings ever crafted by man. The magnanimous sounds and smells of the natural world float upon a stagnant pocket of carbon monoxide and cigarette smoke, while the jungle slowly envelops the empty packs and casually discarded soda cans.

When walking on the side of the road, you have a choice of what to see. On one side there is the ubiquitous pervasion of human filth, spewed forth unto the world as if it were God's plan. On the other side is the forgotten beauty everyone races past every morning in their immortal haste to escape their vehicle; their wonderfully constructed chariot which carries them wherever their heart desires, with whatever music they choose to hear heralding their triumphant conquest of the jerk in the car next to them.

I really try hard to only see one world, the world which sits on top of the perversion. The world the birds see, not the indiscriminant litterings of our precious modern age. While I lived in Edgewater I walked everywhere I went for eight years. Most of the places I went were not serviced by the sidewalk, only by the highway. It seems like a normal place to walk, but for some reason somewhere along the way, the sidewalk ends, and the path ahead is no longer painstakingly paved for your leisurely perusal. You never see any other person walking these routes, but on a regular basis you would see me, walking through the rain with an overloaded backpack full of groceries, and every available limb swinging bags of produce.

It would take me sometimes an hour to psych myself up for one of these journeys. I wear isolation headphones so that the insults and provocations of the ever charming humans wouldn't reach my ears. Sometimes they did. Why I have to spend hours trying to console myself because of some offensive nonsense some moron yells out the window of their automobile is beyond me. I look only into the enveloping arms of nature which seemingly everyone else has ignored.

Despite my efforts, the insidious attacks of my fellow man sometimes spoils the serenity. To be completely happy while walking in the rain is an art form in and of itself. I perfected the craft, but just then the side mirror of a car glanced by my ear. It was a redneck in an oversized pickup truck trying to drive through the massive puddle I was stepping through and splash me. They lost control and smashed their mirror on a street sign a few feet in front of me as the vehicle bounced up onto the curb.

For anyone who enjoys this particular pastime, let me just spoil it for you right now. It is not difficult to soak someone on their way to work on the side of the road with your car in the rain, but don't you ever brag about it in public because acting on the behalf of all the unfortunate souls doomed to find their way by walking these roads, and in some small part for myself, I will un-regrettably be happy to stealthily throw my ice-water in your face so you too may experience the fun.

I had a few music teaching jobs while I lived in Edgewater. I teach guitar, drums, piano, keyboard, clarinet, bass guitar, and saxophone. Moderately humiliating was taking a cab to work which costs thirty dollars each way, totaling sixty dollars per day, which amounted to half of my income. Even more humiliating was walking to work just down the block everyday where everyone could see me getting run off the side of the road by a tsunami throwing ignoramus in a Chevy, all the while wondering if it was the father of the kid I was walking through the rain to teach. Somehow I put my head down and continued on, and I still music teach today.

I apologize for ranting, I'm clearly bitter about the freedom of others to go where they please, and their insistence to mock me from their climate controlled comfort, or even worse yet friends who call you a homebody (as if you have a choice). It's amazing what hurtful things people will say in their attempts to get a laugh from a group.

When I first moved to Edgewater I spent a lot of time with my brother. Tom is a remarkably consistent person in his hesitance to care about much of anything. I mean this in the most endearing way. He is the kind of person who moves on instantly. I guess you could say he lives in the moment (certainly not the past, maybe occasionally in the future). We spent a lot of time fishing and drinking. He eventually made a full-time job out of the former. The days of sunshine and simple patience required for fishing were really good for me. I could spend hours just thinking through the hard times I'd had, and making my peace with them. We don't go fishing much anymore as I no longer live downstairs like some basement dwelling piano troll. I cherish those years; we had a lot of good fun without much needing to be said.

I practiced the piano often as much as six hours a day while I lived with my brother. We heard of a teacher in Baltimore who had worked at the Baltimore School for the Blind. I went to audition for him, and he accepted me on the condition that my technique be improved first and foremost. John Beyers can trace his teaching lineage back to Franz Liszt, who is considered to be the most famous pianist to have ever lived. Liszt taught Carl Reinecke, who taught Ferruccio Busoni, who in turn taught Mieczyslaw Munz, and Munz taught my teacher, John Beyers.

I had always been the kind of player whose brain made up for his hands. I was able to grasp an entire piece very well, and offer a convincing performance, but there would always be missing details along the way because I never practiced. That all changed during my time with Mr. Beyers.

We'd spend an hour playing scales, arpeggios, and chords of every variety. We harmonized in thirds and sixths, contrary motion and everything. What made the technical practice fruitful is that Mr. Beyers played along with me the entire time. A 70 year old man blazing through harmonic minor scales harmonized at the tenth with contrary motion really puts you in your place. There was no doubt he meant it when he said technique is important. He would painstakingly teach me classical music; I never read a single note off the paper (I couldn't read at all at the time).

We played Tchaikovsky's Piano Concerto No. 1 (with the hard cadenza), Chopin's Revolutionary Etude, Heroic Polonaise, and Ballade No. 1, Liszt's Tarantelle and Mephisto's Waltz, Beethoven's Appasionata Sonata, Rachmaninoff's Prelude in Gm, and Variations on a theme by Corelli.

In 2003 I won first place in the Hinda Honickman competition with a taped performance of the Beethoven Op. 57. Perhaps it took winning a competition for me to give up on competition as a whole. Either way, I'm very proud of what we accomplished, and eternally grateful to Mr. Beyers for sharing his time with me.

Around 2004 I enjoyed a slight recovery of sight in the focal point of my left eye. It is about the size of a pinhead, but the placement is impeccable, making it possible for me to read again. Many with LHON refer to this small area of vision as a "sweet spot." This allows me to read about one word at a time and to focus on a small object in the distance. Eight years into the recovery I won't say it drastically changed anything, but I was able to return to school.

Over 3 years I earned an Associate's degree at the Anne Arundel Community College. I paid my own way every semester and I took the bus roundtrip every day for classes, and taught music lessons in the evenings. The college is only a 15-minute drive from where I lived, but on the bus it took an hour and fifteen minutes to get there! The ride home was only 45 minutes. So to go to a college which was right down the street, I paid $12 a day bus fare, and made a 2-hour commute. I took my time while I was at the campus as you can imagine. I took many varied classes in music, science, and math (my favorite subjects). I'd spend 2 hours just playing piano in one of the practice rooms to kill time until my next class.

The main thing I learned from this time paying my own tuition and making a ridiculous commute was that I could take control of my own life, but it wouldn't be easy. It became clear to me that none of the adversity in my life would likely disappear. People will always mock me for walking wherever I go as an adult. People will always insinuate that I don't work as hard as they do because I leave my Fridays open in case I need to reschedule lessons. People will always expect me to be able to do something simple like recognize them, even though it's physically impossible for me to do.

One time someone who recognized me from high school actually pushed me up against a wall and taunted me. He said, "You don't even know who I am" and laughed. I've learned that my path will always be harder than the person next to me, and some will do anything they can to belittle me, or to make they feel like they work harder.

Then you have old friends whose only desire is to chastise you for your inability to effectively cope with going blind, as if they'd have done so much better. Then there are those who just have the story wrong all together, and of course they are the ones who talk the most, spreading misinformation about you all over town as if it were their business in the first place. I find the people who talk the most say the least, and hear the least as well, and I'm not interested in talking to people who do not listen.

There are people who make everything a competition: what a miserable lot! There are things in this world that are ubiquitous and beautiful (music comes to mind) and these bastards make a competition out of it. They take something beautiful and turn it into something ugly. A lot of jazz musicians are guilty of this in my experience. Instead of appreciating that they get to improvise music and get paid for it, they turn it into how many songs they know compared to you, how fast can you play, or can you use an altered scale? For a moment let me boast and say that I can play a lot of difficult music at a fast tempo, on at least ten different instruments and in countless idioms, but I would never make any other musician feel bad for not being able to do so. My friend David Zee put it well, saying "it's not a race, it's art!"

My favorite music is intuitive, simple, and organic. It doesn't ask or require anything of you, it just gives you pleasure. That's how it should be! So literally every time someone tries to make a competition out of a simple conversation, I just walk away.

I wish I could take credit for this philosophy, but it comes from a classic Chinese book I read with my newly revised vision, a book which definitely changed my life, Tao Te Ching. The line in particular that has become my mantra when someone is telling me they're better than me or they work harder is, "In not competing you are without competition." So simple, so beautiful, so useful!

While in Edgewater, the Leber's disorder of my family began to appear among my sister Valerie's kids. My nephew Chase began to suffer a loss of vision at age six. Valerie became a real guru with the ins and outs of the disease, and all the research offering hope on the horizon. She was able to keep me informed of new developments in research, as I was too busy trying to claw my way through my own life.

Chase has always been a bright child. He was well equipped to deal with this unfortunate turn of events. I didn't have a lot of experience with children at this time: to be honest they made me nervous. I feel like I was not able to assist Chase very well in finding his way with the disease. I had no great secrets to share, only bitterness. I hoped my solidarity and silent strength would be assistance enough, but I wish I had talked to him more about what was happening. Somehow, without my help he did just fine adjusting.

A few years later, my younger nephew Grant began to show a vision loss as well at age eight. Again, my lack of relation to the mindset of youth prevented me from being very helpful to my young nephew, but luckily there are now people in the world who are much more helpful than I could have ever hoped to be. Grant has undertaken an incredible journey with this disease, no pun intended, considering he has to constantly travel to across the country to see Dr. Sadun in California. His experience is the final chapter of this book. Grant is a very brave young man for taking all those cross-country trips with his mother, and spending so much time at the doctor's office. Imagine such a pioneer at such a young age! It is very inspiring.

We were able to heal together as a family was through music. I taught my nephews and my niece a variety of instruments over the years: piano, guitar, and clarinet. During our time Chase achieved some great milestones—he even performed all three movements of the Moonlight Sonata. I hope that my solidarity and consistency in teaching them music served them better than fleeting words of reassurance could have during their hardship. They are great kids, and I love my sister's family very much.

My time at the edge of the water taught me to take control of my life, and to ignore the petty attacks of friends and strangers. It also was a time spent waiting to find the right person to share my life and home with. I dated some unfortunate creatures during this time, but in the end my unpaved path led me right where I want to be.

Pride in where I am today (2009—)

"How did I stumble into this room?
I saw a face
In triumph of all the comfortable human pain
I clamped my eyes open
And stumbled into a fantastic room

There is a painting of a lute on the wall
Tears fall whenever I see it
I stare blankly into the face of God
There is life all around

I am still surrounded by the splendid face
That drew me here
Outside my everything
Inside the vibrations

I was overgrown by your eyes a thousand times
Before I noticed they encompass all
And have held me close
For longer than I ever dreamed."

-Larry Byrne, "Living Room", 2012

I no longer live in the basement of a townhouse. My wife Jenn and I own a beautiful home in Maryland. It sits on a half acre of land which boasts dense forest, arid grassland, low swamp, evergreens, and a vast garden (It's got a little bit of everything!).

I met Jenn Reichwein through a piano student who played with a band called the Hypnotic Panties. I'd go to see them play, and end up getting roped in to help them fix a sound problem. I started talking with Jenn, who plays guitar and sings with the group. I always liked her sense of humor. There was one time I went to see them on a hot July day and the air conditioning was broken at the bar they were playing. I don't remember exactly what she said, but I remember her making light of the extreme heat, and just generally having a good attitude about it. We'd occasionally see each other and we always enjoyed each other's conversation, although we did not start dating for many years.

Jenn works as a programmer for the DC3 Cyber Crime Center, so she is up early every day. On a Tuesday in May 2008 the air conditioning was broken at her house. She took the day off on Wednesday to wait for the repairman, and headed out for a rare Tuesday night on the town. One of our local heroes here in Annapolis is Jimmy Haha, from Jimmie's Chicken Shack.

He also has a group called the Jarflys who were performing at Armadillos that night. I too went out for a rare Tuesday outing to see the Jarflys. I ran into Jenn, who I had not seen for quite a while, and we chatted all night. I gave her a big hug when we parted ways, and found that I continued to think about her for days after.

I worked up my nerve to ask her out at a big music festival, Eastport-a-Rockin', where we were both performing. She did not respond and ran off towards a nearby tent. I thought perhaps I had offended her or made her feel nervous. Next thing I knew she was pulling a toddler out of an ice bin into which he had fallen into head first. There was a big commotion; obviously she had just saved the child's life. After all that excitement she agreed to go out with me, and apologized for running off, but I think we are all glad she did!

Jenn introduced me to the world of Bluegrass music. I had never heard it before meeting her. The world of acoustic music and old-time melodies instantly grabbed me and I've spent a lot of time studying it ever since. There are superstars in Bluegrass, but in general it is a very humble and accepting music. A 20-year recording and performing veteran can stand and play in a jam next to a hobbyist housewife, and both of them are elated to be playing the music they love. There are not many forms of music these days that really unite people in such a way.

Jenn's father Pete Reichwein is a well-known figure in the Bluegrass community (although he is not a Bluegrass-only player) and he has really developed a unique style on the Dobro. With our family trio we even play Brazilian jazz tunes like Tico Tico and he plays the melody on the Dobro! I love being able to play music with my wife, and I only wish we had more time to do it!

Most of my time these days is spent teaching and playing music (as always!). I teach at the School of Rock Annapolis, where I get to work with a large group of really nice kids. I have private students on piano, guitar, bass, and banjo, and I direct shows three times a year. The last two were British Invasion and Motown. We work with the kids for 3 to 4 months and then they perform two concerts to wrap it all up. It's a great program; I wish they had something like that when I was young.

Music is obviously my world. I learned the piano, saxophone, and clarinet in my youth. I taught myself to play the guitar, banjo, mandolin, cuatro, bass guitar, violin, drums, upright bass, and harmonica. The other large chunk of my time goes to the band, Higher Hands. I met Jason Crawford of the band probably around 2003, and we have worked together in some capacity ever since. Higher Hands is an unusual group in that we have no stringed instruments. I play left hand bass on the keyboard for all the selections.

When I started running baselines, which are the low-pitched instrumental parts used in several styles of popular music, there were not any good sounds on the keyboards available. I happened to have a Roland Fantom X6 workstation synthesizer keyboard which has a built in sampler. I took my wife's Fender Precision Bass and recorded every note on it, from E to C on the 4th string, then 4 chromatic notes up the 3rd and 2nd strings, and then from Bb all the way up the neck on the 1st string. I had to expand the sampler memory on the Fantom, but I was able to load all the recorded notes into the keyboard and assign them to a specific key.

Anybody who has done this knows that the synthesizer doesn't automatically sound like a bass guitar: it sounds pretty horrible. The Fantom offers some really advanced filters so in effect the harder you hit a key, the brighter the note sounds. I created my bass patch in one day. A bass patch is a combination of filters and recordings that allow the synthesizer to actually sound like a bass guitar. It was 13 hours of fiendish work, but I have not had to modify the filters or samples to this day.

The Higher Hands plays a really eclectic form of music; it really defies explanation. There is jazz in it, there is R&B in it, there is Go-go (Washington, D.C. Go-go that is), there is hip-hop, there is reggae—in short it is a band with an identity crisis. All the players in the group are phenomenal, and that's what allows us to blend such a varied concoction of styles in a convincing manner. We are releasing our second record entitled "Stay Sharp" as of November 17, 2012. We perform A LOT, especially during the summer months, so it's not uncommon for me to work a full week teaching and play six gigs in a week. I suppose it is good to stay busy.

I love to cook although I don't have much time for it. I work until either 9:00pm or 2:00am every night except an occasional Tuesday or Sunday, but when I can, I really enjoy the creative process of making a fantastic meal. I especially love when all the ingredients are grown right in my own garden. It is so rewarding to enjoy the healthy goodness of fresh homegrown vegetables!

Standing where I am today at my house on, both figurative and literally, Pride Lane, it is hard to relate back to those dark days when my vision loss first happened to me. There is still a lot of bitterness; I definitely have a chip on my shoulder when it comes to certain things. I still remember certain pains, and when I think of them I am inconsolable. Despite it all I am still able to face each day with optimism, and hope. I try not to let the past despicable acts of some ruin my future opinion of most. My days are filled with music of all kinds, and I have my lovely wife, and our pets Django, Bunky, and Jose to share them with. I am very happy, which is not something I would have said at many points along the way. I am very thankful to my mother and father, my brother and sister and her family, all of my close friends, and my wife, Jenn.

So I live, as Candide, a hopeless optimist with an ever growing Tsunami hot on my heels. I maintain that if our species would generally speak less and do more, act less selfishly, and treat each other as leaves of the same tree (which we are), we could all enjoy the marvelous beauty which has been laid out before us, simple as that.

"Beneath the River's constant weary flow
Her unending motion, it don't always show
Upon the Mountain there is no sound
This ain't no time for singing, ain't no birds around.
On down the River, my final bed
She coldly watch me, my grim old friend
So into the Water we proudly fall
We take nothing with us so we know we have it all

On down the Highway we coil and bend
Days feel like nothing and nights have no end
On the wide Horizon dark clouds a-form
I got a bad, bad feeling, man it's gonna pour
But into the fury we cast our gaze
Hope we want for nothing at the end of our days

When faith is slim, and all around is wrath
Remember that the Water never seeks to change its path

Own less to have more
Speak less and do more
Flow like a River to the nearest Sea
Cause the more you want
The more you need"

-Larry Byrne, "The Path", 2010

http://higherhandsmusic.com/

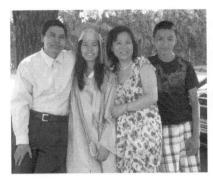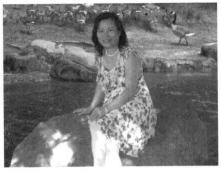

A Second Chance

I can do everything through Him who gives me strength.

Philippians 4:13

When I was five years old, the Khmer Rouge captured Cambodia and forced all city residents into the countryside. The Khmer Rouge was the communist guerilla group led by Pol Pot. Since my family lived in the city, we were forced to evacuate. Through these hard times, I also had to bear the loss of my mother.

After walking through what is today referred to as the Killing Fields, I realized I was losing my vision. This happened during the night when it was extremely dark and there was no light to guide us. I suddenly realized I couldn't see from my left eye and the world around me soon became darker. I cried for help, but no one heard me. There were no doctors around; everyone was busy fighting for their own lives. Scared of what was happening, I told my dad I couldn't see. He brushed it off as if it was no big deal, and didn't believe me.

Often I would sit on a roadside staring at the sky, cradling my pounding head in my hands. "This blurry vision had better go away by early morning," I told my dad. In order to survive, I had to keep on walking—without any shoes on my feet. I was dying of hunger and thirst, but moving forward was necessary. As hard as it was, I knew deep down that I was going to make it.

175

My family and I arrived safely in the United States on October 28, 1981, with a new identity. I did not speak a word of English; my clothes were all patched and torn.

I grew up visually impaired, which is not easy. Everyone around me thought that I was perfectly normal, but they didn't know the real me. Growing up with my dad and five sisters, but they had no idea what was going on in my life. They never came to the conclusion that I couldn't see. Many times I tried to explain yet, they didn't take the time to listen. It seemed as though they didn't care.

I had a dysfunctional family growing up; I was physically and emotionally abused. Everyone was so busy with their own lives, so how would they notice my issues? How can they take care of me when they can't even take care of themselves? As a result, I had to learn to get through things on my own. As much as I wanted someone to be there for me, I was alone in this darkened world.

During elementary school, I remember when I took my first vision exam at the family doctor's office; my left eye failed completely. At that point my dad took me to an ophthalmologist, and again failed the test. The doctor asked me about my family history, when I had lost my vision, and was I exposed to anything. I told the ophthalmologist everything, but he had no clue what the problem might be. The doctor prescribed me glasses and said I probably lacked nutrition when I was in Cambodia.

Once the doctor had confirmed my left eye lacked vision, some of my sisters said, "I don't understand you. You are so good at school, smart, and you can drive. You are in track, tennis, and in choir." And a few of the sisters would add, "You're just pretending so you can slack off." No one can honestly say they would choose to live the life that I have had. My sisters don't understand how hard it has been for me to be the person I am. I may have made it seem easy, but each day was a struggle. Often I wanted to give up, but I knew that wasn't the right thing to do. In the long run everything I worked for would all be worth it. I was a fighter.

My sisters had no idea how their comments were tearing me up inside. They made me feel as though I was lying and couldn't do anything. All this time I had been trying to earn acceptance from my family and all they did was discourage me. They would continually discourage me and make me feel worthless.

I kept my personal feelings to myself. Through my strong willed personality, I would pretend nothing was wrong, even during the times I was falling apart. When I wanted to do something, I was determined to do it. I had felt that I was a unique person since I was five years old, yet I tried to live my life as normal as possible. When other people read or wrote things, the same tasks would take me longer to do. I never had extra time or any assistance in my classes. I was in regular classes just like everyone else. After school, while other people were playing, I had to study.

I was striving to be a perfectionist. My visual impairment was never noticed. I don't remember growing up classifying myself as "blind." I fooled so many other people; I even ended up fooling myself thinking that I was normal.

I graduated from Hoover High School with good grades, but I still could not gain my father's attention. I remember I received straight A's when I was a freshman. I showed my dad, but he did not bother to look. I worked during the summer and gave him all my money. I was an obedient child, but I was still rejected. I had hopes of gaining my dad's love and a strong desire for him to be proud of me. I was the first one out of six siblings to get to be able to go to California State University Fresno. Out of his six daughters, I am the only one who is visually impaired. I wanted my dad to embrace me and tell me, "I am proud of you, Phoeng," and to accept me for who I am as a daughter, not as a son. From this day forward, I know I cannot change my dad. Only my dad himself can change that. I'm going to take one step at a time and enjoy each moment at a time.

Shortly after graduating from high school, I married my wonderful husband, Paul Gip. Being married was not as great as I had dreamed. Being married sure has its ups and downs, but it is all a part of life. At the age of 20 I had my first child, Michell. And five years later, I had a son, Matthew. And on top of all that, Paul and I had a successful business together. Life was going great up to this point.

In the summer of 2003 things started to change, and not for the better. Most summers, I had enjoyed taking my kids everywhere with me. We could spend quality time together. It was then that I noticed Matthew's vision wasn't good. As he would try to read a newspaper he had to put it close to his face. I knew this wasn't normal. I tried not to panic and decided to schedule an eye doctor's appointment for both of my kids.

After the checkup, we learned that Matthew was nearly legally blind in one eye. Michell had lost some vision, but we didn't think much of it. We had no idea what was going on, but hoped nothing would get any worse from this point on. At 5 years old, it was difficult to know what his vision was like. By observing him, I knew his vision was getting worse. He told me it was too blurry and fuzzy. I knew this was a not good sign. As for Michell, her grades started to drop, she had several missing assignments, and low test scores. Earlier, she had always excelled. I knew something was very wrong.

We went to doctor after doctor with the hope of finding out what was going on. At the same time, I was afraid of finding out something terrible. I had no idea what it could be, but I was hoping there would be a cure. I would do anything for my children. It wouldn't matter how much it cost or how far I would have to go. I couldn't bear seeing my children go through all this pain and suffering.

One doctor told us that Michell may have a brain tumor since her vision was deteriorating so rapidly. We quickly did as many tests as possible. I wanted to know that it wasn't something as severe as a brain tumor, since that could be deadly. I was thinking the worst, but hoping for the best. Finally we went to a genetic doctor and found out what was happening. "We've determined what's causing their vision loss," she said. She hesitated, then continued, "They have Leber's Hereditary Optic Neuropathy (LHON)."

At the age of 31, at the same time as my children, I was diagnosed with Leber's Hereditary Optic Neuropathy. I never knew my vision loss could be hereditary. I was devastated. I became extremely depressed and lonely. I gave up driving and cried myself to sleep each night.

The self-esteem and assertiveness that I once enjoyed grew less with each passing day, replaced by silence. My children suffered even worse than me, and each became legally blind. I had worked so hard to plan out their futures and now my dreams were shattered to pieces

When we received the diagnosis, my heart sank. What? LHON? Me? No way! I was a healthy person. Impossible! Why, out of all of my sisters, was I the only who couldn't see? Why me and both of my children? I can't believe this. Life is not fair.

I didn't accept it. "No!" I insisted. "Matthew is 5 years old and Michell is 10 years old. That must be a mistake."

"I wish it were," the genetic doctor said. "They can take Carnitine daily. Also they can do a procedure using Carnitine plus IV injections once a week for three months with the hope to prevent any further vision loss and hope to restore some vision back. But we must do this procedure immediately and it is extremely expensive."

I didn't know what to say or think, but I was willing to take that chance for my children, so of course we would try. But, I was lost and confused. I had hit rock bottom in my life. I had no one to turn to for support. From that moment on, I became so emotional I had to seek some counseling.

The genetic doctor's words seemed muffled, distant, like when you're waking up from a nightmare. But this was no nightmare. This was my harsh reality. And no matter how much money I invested in my children's treatments, I couldn't find a cure. Money become meaningless: I wanted my children to see.

Unfortunately, the procedure did not go well and brought more bad news. My children were blind and they would have to learn Braille and Orientation and Mobility. They had to transfer from an upscale school to a downscale school. Michell went from a straight A student to an F student. It was one thing for me to have lost my vision, but that pain paled in comparison to the loss of my children's eyesight.

I needed to inform this horrific news to my extended family, but I didn't know how. I am one of the Khmer Rouge survivors from 1975-1979, I could do this. Over the next couple of days I nervously told my extended family.

"How'd the appointment go?" asked my dad, clearly expecting good news. My silence told him otherwise.

"What is it?" he asked.

I bit my quivering lower lip in an effort to keep from crying. "I . . . I got some bad news," I told him. "It's LHON," I said, almost in a whisper.

He remained silent and motionless. And he said to me that when it comes to bad news, he has to hear it first. When it comes to good news, no one tells him.

Some of my sisters would say, "You can still drive, all you have to do is pull your car a little closer to the sign. If you can read a book, how can you say that you are blind?" they questioned me. "And your eyes look good." Hearing their comments certainly didn't help me feel any better. I was looking for some kind of comfort, but surely I wasn't going to get that from my extended family.

Later, I returned to the genetic doctor's office for a routine checkup for my children. When the doctor entered, she looked at me and began, "Phoeng, I have some news . . ."

My heart skipped a beat.

"I'm afraid your family has no cure or any type of treatment here in the United States," she said. "No need to come back for checkups anymore."

I felt like my stomach was turning upside down. I felt so hopeless and filled with despair. I fell back into the chair, horrified, terrified, and completely confused.

"This doesn't make sense," I cried from my heart.

I felt sick. I closed my eyes and took a deep breath. How will I get through this? Then my competitive instincts kicked in. Come on, you can handle this! I told myself. You are a fighter. Don't back out now! But this was harder than any task, because this was about my children whom I gave birth to.

I prayed, "Please help me, God. I'm really scared. Are my kids destined to be this way? Please Lord; give me strength to go on. Help my kids to restore their vision. I cannot do this all alone."

Tears rolled down my face. I was expecting some kind of comfort at least and some kind of encouraging words, but there were none. I was hoping someone would offer me a ride or sit beside me to listen to me or to give me a shoulder to lean on. But no one did. In general, it is difficult to rely on others, especially for a ride. It is extremely inconvenient. When others had needed my help, I was always there to give them full support, financial or physical. Apparently, the same was not true if I was the one in need of help.

If I had known long ago that I had LHON I don't think I would have wanted any children. It is not that I don't love my children: it is that I can't bear to see the hardships that my children have to go through. Ultimately, I have not once regretted having my children because they have given me so much joy and purpose.

Things happen in life. Good things happen as well. People say they see the healing hand of God in events like the ones in this exchange:.

"Phoeng, there's something I've been meaning to tell you," my sister said. "You're the strongest person I know. After watching you, I've learned that anything is possible and you've taught me to have faith. No matter what life throws at me, I know I can overcome it and become a stronger person. I know that from watching you."

My sibling words humbled me. "Don't be so impressed," I said. "I used to take God for granted. It was like I knew He was there, and that seemed to be enough. But when my children became blind, I became a Christian and I prayed more. As my body grew weaker, my spirit grew stronger. And I'm never alone."

"Were you ever angry with God?" one sibling asked.

"I was at war with blindness, not with God," I said. "How could I be mad at Him? God knows that I'm a stubborn person; He was using my children to turn my life around. He gave me a new perspective on life. I may be physically blind, but I'm no longer spiritually blind. I have a second chance to relive my life. Besides, I get to experience both worlds: a sighted world and a blind world, one with each eye. My eye may be blind, but inside my heart I can see so clearly."

"Are you scared that your right eye would go blind too?"

"Yes! If I told you no, I would be lying to you. But I am almost 38 years old now. I don't want to waste my time worrying about something that may or may not happen," I said. "Besides, God wants me to live for today by appreciating and using the gifts I have now. And that's precisely what I'm going to do." All I can do is not to give up, not lose hope, and continue to pray for my children and for our vision to get better.

God is so good. He gave me these precious children because He knows I am capable and strong. I enrolled myself in Fresno City Community College and received my AS degree in Business Management in fall 2010. There is nothing a visually impaired person cannot do; except the driving part. Nothing is impossible if you are willing and have determination.

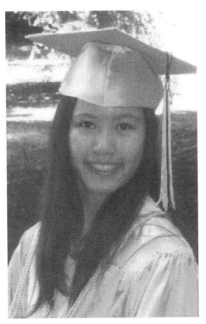
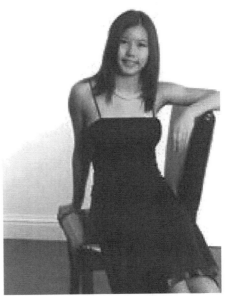

The Life Unexpected
By Michell Gip

Tough times don't last, but tough people do (Norman Vincent). In life, people always have to go through struggles and hard times. Those times don't last forever, but the way you handle it will forever stick with you. Sometimes, you may th ink you know a person, but no one really knows what they've had to go through. Everyone has their own experiences that are both good and bad. In my own life, I have had many struggles, but have learned to realize that it what has made me who I am today.

My early elementary school years were as normal as any other child's. I had a good family and was lucky enough to go to a good school. I made a lot of friends, and for the most part actually enjoyed going to school. Initially, I was shy around people I didn't know, but after I knew a person, I was pretty social.

Throughout the years, I started becoming more active in school, such as joining choir, basketball, the school play, and cheerleading, all while managing to be one of the top students in the class. I thought I had it all, and nothing would stop me from being the best of the best.

As I look back, most people would tell me that I was self-centered and acted as if I was stuck up. In my mind, I knew I was good at what I did, and just wanted everyone to know it. This attitude showed through my actions and people didn't like that. But then I reached the summer before fifth grade. I thought it would be a great year of cheer and basketball, but little did I know that this school year was going to change my life forever.

The summer before my fifth grade year, my parents thought it would be a good idea for me to have an eye doctor's appointment. I figured there would be nothing to it, since my vision seemed perfectly fine. I went and found out my left eye wasn't as good as my right, so they told me I had a lazy eye and prescribed me glasses. It was no big deal because many kids wore glasses. It wasn't as if I was going to be an outcast or anything.

A few months after school started, I noticed I wasn't able to read the board or even papers right in front of me, with or without my glasses. Teachers thought I was probably crazy or just didn't want to do the work. I was scared of what was happening and didn't know what to do. Each day, my vision was slowly disappearing right before my very own eyes.

We went to an eye specialist in town and did all the testing we could to see what was going on. The hardest part was waiting for the results, but no one knew anything. At this point I wasn't able to read the board, any text in front of me, or continue any extra-curricular activities at school. Life as I knew it was changing, yet there wasn't anything I could do about it.

Finally, on November 15, 2003, I was diagnosed with Leber's Hereditary Optic Neuropathy (LHON). It is a rare genetic eye disease that causes a loss of central vision and would leave me legally blind. Doctors told me there was nothing I could do about it and just learn to accept it. I heard what everyone was telling me, but it was all a blur. I just couldn't accept the fact that I would have to live like this for the rest of my life. This was a nightmare, and I hoped I would wake up soon. But I realized I was living this nightmare and couldn't get out of it, so this ended up being the worst day of my life.

184

My parents didn't accept this diagnosis at first either. Being their only daughter, it must have been heartbreaking for them. It wasn't something that we talked about much, but I knew it affected everyone in the family. Not only was this happening to me, but my brother was also going through the same struggle. My younger brother, Matthew, was only five at the time. I could not even imagine what he might have been going through himself. Nor could I imagine how my parents have felt watching both of their kids go legally blind. My parents wanted to do anything they could, but doctors kept saying there wasn't any type of treatment or cure.

I kept hearing the doctors' words ringing in my head. I just couldn't believe this was happening to me; out of all people, why me? I had such a big family, and why did both my brother and I have to be affected? It just didn't make any sense to me. I didn't think I deserved this harsh punishment. Life was just cruel, and I hated it! I felt as though no one knew what I could possibly be going through.

My family and I didn't listen to the doctors' words, though. We were determined to find some sort of treatment. A few weeks after being diagnosed, we decided I should take Carnitine. It was supposed to help the optic nerves. Unfortunately, I didn't show any signs of improvements after a few months. So the doctors suggested I take the Carnitine through an IV once a week. They said it would help it go through my system quicker and therefore show quicker signs of improvements. The only problem with this was that it was extremely expensive. No matter how expensive, though, my parents were willing to do anything to help me get my vision back.

After three months of taking the Carnitine through an IV, I still showed no signs of improvements. I had this hollow feeling when I heard the doctors' words. In hopes of gaining some improvements, I still took the Carnitine for another year. I was in denial of what was going on, but didn't want to give up yet. I knew this was a battle, and I couldn't let this disease defeat me. I've never been known to give up before, so I couldn't give up now.

After realizing that the Carnitine wasn't doing much if anything, I stopped taking it. I didn't know what else to do. School was harder than ever. Everything I enjoyed doing had to stop. All of my friends started treating me differently. Some of my extended family acted as if I was contagious. It

185

was just an out-of-control world that I was living in. I felt as though no one understood me. I was all alone in this world that I no longer knew. Nothing was familiar to me was there anymore. It was all changing and I didn't know how to handle it.

As if things weren't bad enough, I found out I would have to transfer schools. My vision was so bad that I had to learn Braille. But the district I was in didn't have a Braille teacher, so I had to go to a school across town. It was inconvenient, but I had no other choice. It was a hard adjustment since I attended an upscale school my entire life. And this school was on a bad side of town where the students were different. I had to learn to overlook that factor and remember my purpose. I was here to learn Braille and adjust to the life as a visually-impaired student.

For a few years after that, my main focus was to do well in school and learn to accept my visual impairment. I tried not to let it bring me down, but life just wasn't the same. I couldn't do all the things I wanted to and students made fun of me constantly. It was a battle among my academic, social, and family life. In the beginning of my eighth grade year, I came to the realization that the quicker I accepted my visual impairment, the quicker people would accept me. Therefore, I tried to make the best of things in life. I worked harder in school, even though it took me longer to read and understand things. I felt like I was slow and stupid sometimes, but knew it wasn't true. Other times, I felt like giving up, but figured that wouldn't be worth it in the end. And I had to learn to join other activities that would work with a visual impairment. For example, I started swimming, playing the piano, and volunteering with children. These things made me happier, and others didn't make fun of me when my confidence started coming back. I try to be as normal as I can be, even with a visual impairment.

As hard as I tried, I still wasn't as happy as I could be. My heart was still in cheer and basketball. I wanted to be like everyone else and do the things that everyone else did. Not only that, I wanted to try to be better. But with a visual impairment, I felt as if that would never happen. I despised the fact that I was now dependent on others. I had to ask for help when I couldn't read something. I couldn't do certain things on my own, which frustrated me. Throughout my life, I was so used to my peers asking me for help and relying on me, and now it was just the opposite.

Everyone constantly told me how strong I was for going through something like this, but none of that mattered to me. I missed who I used to be and couldn't get it out of my mind. All of my hopes and dreams for the future were crushed. It tore me up inside, this life I had to live in. No one knew it, even the people closest to me. I would remember crying from all the sadness and frustration, and voices all around would tell me to stop. I just figured it wasn't right to cry, so I stopped. I kept everything to myself, and didn't want anyone to know all the pain I was in.

Each day I went to school and put on a smile. I laughed at everyone's jokes. For the most part, I tried to be outgoing. It wasn't always easy, but I tried. I knew this wasn't the real me. I don't know why I kept pretending. I didn't know how to express my emotions to those I love. I bottled myself up ready to explode. Behind my smile and laughter, all I wanted to do was cry.

Despite my emotional instability, I strived to be who I used to be. It seemed impossible, but in my mind it was possible. I started high school at Clovis North High School. It was a new school and I was ready to make traditions and start legacies. Being the first visually-impaired student at Clovis North, I wanted to be someone whom future students would remember. I wanted to be their inspiration, someone they could look up to for future reference.

In high school, I took many rigorous classes. Teachers and administrators all told me I was unable to take those classes because it would be too challenging, especially since I had a visual impairment. It discouraged me at first, but eventually made me more motivated. I wanted to prove them wrong. Because of my stubbornness and strong-willed personality, I wouldn't take no for an answer. Eventually, I got the classes I wanted and excelled.

After about five years of being diagnosed with LHON, I was more confident and comfortable with myself. I can't honestly say I was happy, but I was OK with how life was going. I decided to do more extra-curricular things in school. I became a part of the community more by volunteering; participating in debates and mock trials, and anything else I could think of. It made me feel a part of something, like my life was before I was diagnosed. People were surprised that I was able to be actively involved as a visually-impaired person.

As if life wasn't crazy enough, I got an unexpected call in late March of 2009. A good friend, Kyle, called me up. The first thing he asked me was, "What eye condition do you have?" I thought it was so random, but answered each one of his questions knowing he had a purpose for asking.

After his questioning, I asked, "Why'd you ask?" He then proceeded to tell me that he'd heard about stem cell research in China. I thought he was just joking around with me since that's the way he is sometimes. He explained to me how a couple of people he knew had just recently come back from the procedure and thought it would be a good idea if I went. He convinced me that it was worth it to take all that time and money to go. In the end it might help my vision. He knew that's what I wanted more than anything in the world: just to have perfect vision again.

As soon as I got off the phone, I eagerly told my parents what Kyle had told me. I looked it up on the Internet as fast as my computer would run. Now that I knew this, I just wanted to know more. I looked up everything possible. For that night, I neglected all homework assignments that I had. I had so many questions, but all the answers couldn't be found in one night.

I was not sure what my parents thought about my new plans, but I honestly thought that they figured I was insane or something. Both of them just had so many questions spiraling through their minds. How much does the stem cell treatment cost? How long does it take? What's the procedure? How many people have gone before me already? Has anyone with LHON ever had it yet? What are the risks? Are there any guarantees? And is it a scam?

The questions were never ending, but I spent numerous hours of research on this. I needed to answer each and every one of their questions with ease. I wanted to assure them that this was safe and the right thing to do. Even though the cost was a ridiculous amount, and I would have to spend a month in China, I thought it would be worth it. And I wanted my parents to feel the same way, since they'd be the one's supporting me. After endless hours of research, my parents finally agreed to let me go to China to undergo this stem cell treatment.

When I'm excited about something, I want to tell everyone. However, I only told the people closest to me, because I knew other people wouldn't understand. Most people don't understand me as is; how would they possibly understand why I feel the need and desire to restore my vision? I was enthusiastic and looking forward to this adventure in my life, but I quickly realized no one else seemed to care or even believe me for that matter. Friends thought I was crazy. Family didn't believe me and told me it was a stupid idea. They kept telling me it was all a scam and not worth it. Hoping to get the most support from those I love, I got the most criticism from them. It was discouraging.

Despite their discouraging comments, my parents were still supportive of me. They knew it was a risk, but were willing to go that extra mile. I didn't have to feel so alone on this journey. No one believed that my family and I were willing to take that kind of risk. They were skeptical and unsure of everything that we had decided on. Now it was just the process of applying, funding the trip, and hoping for the best.

My mom was worried of everything that could happen if I were to go to China. She told me that she'd rather be the one to go first and see what the procedure was like. Therefore if anything were to go wrong, it would happen to her and not her children. But, I already had my heart set on going to China in hopes of restoring my vision. I'd wanted this for so long, my mom wouldn't be the one to stop me from going now. I listened to what she had to say and took all of her arguments into consideration. That didn't convince me though. When my parents felt they were ready to fill out the initial application for the treatment, I put my name on the application instead.

It was a matter of days before I received an email stating that I was approved for stem cell treatment in China. This process was all done through email and my parents weren't that familiar with technology at that time. I was the one who had to fill everything out. As I was filling out the initial application, I knew my mom wanted me to fill it out with her name instead, but I didn't want to. She was disappointed when she found out what I had done, but realized there wasn't anything she could do about it. So from that point on, it was all about getting ready to go to China.

Life was so hectic; I wasn't sure how I was going to keep up with everything. This was the middle of the semester with midterms, AP studying, and everything else. Going to China was just another thing I had to do. I spent endless hours reading about other people's experiences, how the procedure went, and watched videos that people had recorded. It assured my family and me that everyone we researched found positive results and had a good experience. My parents still had a fear of it being a scam. They said, "They can still pay people to write blogs and make videos." It was just hard to tell since you weren't able to talk to the person, except via email. And for things like that, there are always a lot of scams.

There was nothing we could do besides pray about the treatment. I constantly thought about it. I thought about all the advantages and disadvantages. We wanted to make sure this was the right thing for me and we wouldn't regret it afterwards. Over time, I told my parents about everything that I found online and they agreed that it was safe and was probably not a scam. But they still wanted to see the costs and all of the details. We went forward with the application process.

A couple weeks later, we found out how long I would have to stay there and how much it all would cost. It came to be $26,300 for six stem cell injections, and would require a one-month stay. I was astonished to find that it was so expensive, but still wanted to go. I didn't think about whether or not my parents were able to afford it or how we would raise the money if we needed to. I knew I was going to China during the summer no matter what. No one and nothing was going to prevent that.

Since my parents owned a small family business dealing with agriculture, they had many vendors for the numerous items that we sold. I told my parents I wanted to write a letter to them asking for a donation. At first my parents thought I was joking. When I had the chance, I wrote a generic letter to all of their vendors, and I showed it to my parents. They were surprised that I would go all out to try and raise some of the money. Surprisingly, their vendors were quite generous and supportive. They seemed more supportive than my own family. Right after sending the letters, I got calls and emails saying they hoped for the best and a check was on the way. I didn't raise a lot of money, but I figured some of it was better than none at all.

Money might have been a big issue, but if so, my parents never told me. They told me not to worry about things like that. They just wanted the best for me. But this time, I wanted to help as much as possible. Since I was in the middle of the semester and busy with so many things, I couldn't do any fundraisers as I had hoped. Somehow when the day to wire the money to China came around, we had enough money. It was a miracle from God I'd like to say, but I'm sure my parents have always been saving money for something like this to happen because I know they wanted my vision restored as much as I did.

In the middle of April, everything was set. We had the date, number of stem cell injections, costs paid for, and everything fell in to place. My mom decided she wanted to be the one to take me. We were set to leave on June 11, 2009, and to come back on July 10, 2009. People at school were counting down the days until the last day of school and so was I, but for a different reason. No one knew that the last day of school would be the start of a whole new adventure for me. My mom and I were going to China together so I could undergo the stem cell treatment. Considering the fact that she's visually impaired in one eye, her vision wasn't all that great either. So it was like the blind leading the blind.

My mom told many more people about the trip than I did. I didn't mind, but people probably thought we were crazy. People were probably thinking how could two visually-impaired people make it to China by themselves? It was definitely going to be a challenge, but we were up for it. Neither of us had traveled before. We had no experience with being in airports. I guess we'd just have to both wait and see what happened. From this point forward, we knew we just had to put everything in God's hands and hope for the best.

The big day was almost here with only four day until we were to leave. We had everything ready and we were just waiting. That day, I got an emergency call from Beike, the stem cell company in China. Beike informed us that we had to relocate to a different city in China. We had been scheduled to stay in Hangzhou, China which was known as a prosperous city. Last minute, they told us we had to go to Qingdao, China. Many Americans were known to go to Qingdao and find it a less modernized city. We didn't particularly want to go there, but Hangzhou was not available because they weren't accepting any foreigners into the city due to the H1N1 virus. Beike paid for our flight rearrangements and worked everything out within 24 hours to make sure we were set.

Thursday, June 11, 2009, finally arrived! I was so excited to go to China. It was my last day of school and right after I would be on my way to China. Just being able to go on this trip has been an emotional roller coaster in itself. It was a challenge to get this far, but I knew it would all be worth it. It was to be a life-learning experience that I'd never forget. No matter what happened during the trip, it would make me a stronger person.

We did everything that they told us; well, as much of it as we could understand. In Hangzhou, they mainly spoke Mandarin, which we don't understand. Our family speaks Cantonese. Beike assured me that someone would be at the airport to pick us up and show us to our next flight to Qingdao. But my mom didn't realize that we had to go to the end of the terminal gate in order for people to wait for us. Since all of this was my idea, I would be the one who was blamed.

My mom didn't see anyone to pick us up and she was getting frustrated. On top of this, she was already exhausted since she wasn't able to sleep much throughout the trip. As we were looking for someone, my mom panics and says, "Where are they, Michell? I thought you said someone would be here to pick us up! What if this is a scam? Where are they?! I don't see anyone." I didn't panic, and just tried to reassure her that we should just walk to the end of the terminal and maybe we'd see people we knew. And once we reached the end, we saw someone holding a sign with my name on it.

We arrived in Qingdao, China, early that Saturday night. As soon as we arrived, we were surprised to meet the doctor right away. Dr. Tony and a translator, Jack, came in to talk to us. When Dr. Tony came in, the first thing he said was, "So, who's the patient here?" It made us laugh because it wasn't obvious who the patient may be. After establishing that the patient was me, Dr. Tony asked us a series of questions regarding our family history of LHON.

Everything started to take off from there. All the testing began with the physical checkups, blood work, and eye appointments. It just all seemed to happen at once, but all of these things had to be done before I would be able to start any of the stem cell injections. Test after test was a different experience in itself. Even taking a cab ride to downtown Qingdao was frightening. The way people drove was different and scary.

After all the testing, the doctors told us I was able to start the stem cell injections. Not only that, but it was also recommended I have acupuncture on a daily basis. It was supposed to help the nerves throughout my body. The first stem cell injections had to be through an IV for safety procedures, in case of an allergic reaction or if anything else were to go wrong. I was so used to IVs, it was a piece of cake. I didn't get any side effects or significant improvements right away. But Dr. Tony said that most people saw more improvements after the spinal. I was scheduled to have my first spinal in a few days.

The spinal is usually a difficult procedure. Younger children who have a spinal are usually put under anesthesia. Since I was slightly older, I got valium, like everyone else. So, it was the day of my spinal. I had read so much about it prior to this day, yet I still was not sure what to expect. My mom and I both prayed, which seemed to ease our nerves.

Jack and another doctor came to tell me that they were ready to start the procedure. Next thing I knew, I was being wheeled into an unfamiliar room. Everything seemed so different than what I was used to. Doctors, nurses, and translators all wore gloves, masks, and other things to keep themselves sanitary. It was strange to see everyone look all different, but I knew it was for my safety. Dr. Tony was there and he was going to be the one to give me my spinal. I had to turn on my side and curl up in a fetal position. They gave me my valium through an IV as promised. A few minutes later I felt all relaxed. I felt as if I didn't care what happened next. I talked to everyone and didn't think about much. I wasn't sure how long it had been, but it didn't bother me because I didn't know what was going on anyway.

The next thing I knew, I heard Dr. Tony telling me it was over. From this point, I would not be able to get up or lift my head for the next six hours. It seemed like a long time at first, but afterwards all I wanted to do was sleep. The first spinal was now done and over with. Somewhere in the room, I heard my mom ask me how things went. I was too tired to even open my eyes, so she just let me sleep.

The next day when the doctors came in, I was still way too tired. They wanted to know how I felt after the spinal and if everything was OK. Now that I had time to think about it, I felt pretty good. I was just exhausted and super sore from lying down for so long. It was definitely a long process. They wanted to know if I thought I had any improvements, but I had to say no at this point. It wasn't like a miracle had happened overnight and now I could suddenly see again. It wasn't magic and I knew that. I just had to patiently wait to see what God had planned for me.

The hardest thing about being in China had to be the waiting. Most of my time was spent waiting. We waited to talk to doctors, for the acupuncture, for the stem cell procedures, and most of all for improvements. Ironically, both my mom and I are the most impatient ones in our family. We were the ones in China anxiously waiting for this miracle to appear before us.

In the morning, as doctors were making their usual visitations, Dr. Tony thought it was time for another eye checkup. According to his records of previous tests, he seemed to have found no change. That didn't bother me much since I'd only had a few treatments. I just figured I would need more time to let the stem cells develop and mature. Therefore, I didn't think much of it, and then he made me switch eyes.

So, now he made me cover my right eye. Every time I cover my right eye I notice my left eye is usually worse; this time was no different. However, it was harder for me to see the letters this time on the eye chart than before the treatment, but I wasn't sure why. I even had Dr. Tony confused and questioning me. I just told him I couldn't read the chart, and he asked me why I didn't show any improvements, as if I would know. It seemed as though I had regressed.

As the afternoon approached, Dr. Tony was ready and eager to do another eye test. He was hoping that this time we would see a difference in my vision and definitely not a decline. If that were to be true, I wouldn't know what to say or do. I had come all this way with hope for improvements, not to find out it's the opposite. That would be heartbreaking to everyone I know and love, but especially for myself. But I knew I couldn't give up hope yet, and I just had to wait and see what the results would turn out to be.

For the second time around, Dr. Tony only wanted to check my left eye since we were having problems with it this morning. I covered my right eye as he instructed and I was surprised to find that I was able to see some of

194

the letters on the eye chart. I knew already that it was better than the test from this morning. In the morning, Dr. Tony had measured 1.3 meters from where I could see the eye chart. But in the afternoon it came to be 2.9 meters. Surprisingly enough, the distance had more than doubled. I didn't realize waiting until the afternoon would make that much difference. This surprised everyone at the hospital, including the doctors, nurses, translators, and all of the other patients. Just having that type of improvement halfway through my treatment didn't seem like a big deal to most people, but to me it was good news. Any news is always better than no news at all. I knew this was just the beginning of something larger. This could be the miracle I've been waiting for. But if not, I'd still had some improvement to make my everyday life better.

In between appointments, we tried to make our time worthwhile. We needed to do something to keep ourselves occupied. I was more of the adventurous type and wanted to explore the city around us. On the other hand, my mom only wanted to do things that were familiar to her. And obviously being in China was not familiar; therefore, at first she preferred to stay in our room and read or go on the computer. She thought I was crazy and felt that it was dangerous. This caused some conflict between us, but there was nothing I could do about it. Eventually people at the hospital convinced my mom that we should go out and explore.

During the week, we only went to places that were nearby. It was nice just to get out of the hospital for awhile. On the weekends, some people in the hospital tried to plan trips together as a group. We went to the beach, a flea market, restaurants, temples, and other tourist attractions.

Everyone always found new places to go and we always wanted to go places. Even though we didn't go to as many places as everyone else, I was the one who always had bad luck. All the strange and unusual things happened to me. One time, we were coming back to the hospital in a cab and got lost. The driver had no idea where he was going and dropped us off at the back of the hospital. It was not like we knew any better, so we just got out and blindly found our way to the right part of the hospital.

After my second IV, I woke up and my finger felt numb. I didn't think much of it, because it has happened before. Throughout the day it started feeling slightly worse. I didn't know whether or not to make a big deal of it. Later that night, my mom and I decided to go out to dinner. While using chopsticks, I realized it hurt when I put the slightest pressure on my finger. Finally I decided to show it to my mom and she confirmed what I already suspected. It was swollen and neither of us knew why.

We went back to the hospital and told the first nurse that we found. The nurse agreed it was swollen and asked if I had gotten bit by anything. As far as I knew nothing had happened. And in the short time getting back, it had gotten worse. The pain ran up my vein on my middle finger. I didn't know what to do nor did I have a clue how it happened. Nurses gave me cream hoping that it would stop the pain. But it didn't go away; it just kept getting worse.

When I woke up the next morning, it wasn't just my finger that was swollen anymore. It now followed one of my veins up to the top of my hand. By the middle of the morning it was up to my arm. This was not a normal side effect from stem cells. We went to find a nurse and doctor to see what was going on, but they didn't seem to know either. They weren't sure whether it was a reaction from the stem cells, acupuncture, or just a bug bite. Dr. Tony couldn't figure out what was wrong so he sent me to a hand doctor and I was put on antibiotics for a week and a half. Over time it healed with no problems, but we never found out the cause of the swelling.

After my last spinal, I was told I had to go to downtown Qingdao to an Eye Institute. This was supposed to be the best Eye Institute in all of Qingdao. I had been there before any of the treatments started and was told go back so that they would have tests for comparison. That Thursday afternoon we made our way downtown.

While I was there, they had my records from before and the doctors said I had better test results this time than the last time, but I wasn't sure how much better. They didn't know how to tell me either, because they didn't speak very much English. In any case, I was just glad that I was showing improvements. I just had to wait for the doctors back at the hospital to evaluate my results and tell me what they thought and what my results were. I would have to wait until the following morning to find out.

Dr. Tony came in the next morning with a few other doctors. He said that the first time I took the visual field test, my central field was most affected from LHON. He said this time it was getting better and it would continue to get better. I was happy to know that my central fields were getting better in both eyes, but my right eye was the one that showed the most improvements.

Dr. Tony also said something that made my mom and I laugh. He said according to the Chinese law I am legally able to drive in China. If anyone has ever been in China, you know what a scary thing that would be. It's like you're unsure if they even have traffic laws.

Secretly I was hoping that I would be able to drive in the United States. It was a few months before my sixteenth birthday and it would have been the best gift of all to know that I could get my license. I would be overwhelmed with happiness to be like everyone and drive a car. I found myself fantasizing about what kind of car I would want and what it would be like to drive.

I really enjoyed the people in the hospital; they were like my stem cell family. We were all there for the same purpose and reason. Either you or a loved one was there to get better for various conditions. We supported each other. No matter how near or far they may be from where I lived, they will forever be close in my heart.

The next day was to be Sunday, July 10, 2009. The end of our China journey had come. It was a trip well spent and would never be forgotten. It was a life learning experience. But it wasn't completely over, as there was still more to come. Early that Sunday morning, we got up and headed to the airport. It was sad to say goodbye to the people we made such good friends with. Not only will I miss the patients, but the supportive staff as well.

Once we arrived in Hangzhou, we had barely enough time to get to the next terminal before our flight was scheduled to leave. We had the fear of missing our flight and the other flight home would then be missed also. This wasn't turning out to be the greatest trip back home. Luckily, we blindly found the right terminal just as everyone was boarding the plane. Catching our breath, we realized we were one flight closer to home, and our next flight would be back to the United States. It was back to California and our regular routines again. And then, wait for the stem cells to improve my vision.

I could have significant or slight improvements. I really wanted to get the most improvement possible. But no matter what, I knew I'd always have my parents to thank for supporting me to go to China. And I'm thankful to God for keeping us safe and helping us each step of the way. We would just have to pray and hope for the best.

Even though the trip was officially over, there was much more to do. From writing my blog and doing an interview video, I was quickly contacted by many people wanting to know more about my experience. Emails came each day asking many questions. Curiosity came from those who wanted to know why we were willing to take such a risk. It was fun getting to meet so many with LHON and having the experience of being able to talk to them.

Everyone had their own opinions as to whether or not it was a good idea for me to go to China. Despite what anyone said I knew it was the right thing for me. The trip was worth the time and money. I wouldn't have changed that for the world. Now I had the opportunity to network with so many others affected by LHON. Some are personally affected and others have family members with LHON. Either way, I was there to talk to them and support them in any way I could. After networking with so many people around the world, I realized my purpose was to inspire and support others.

Speaking to those with LHON has made me become a stronger person. It has taught me not to pity myself, but instead always remember to lend a helping hand to others. The world does not revolve around me: there are many others around me who are suffering

My friends and family informed me about it a few years after I was diagnosed with LHON that I blink much more often than most people. It didn't hurt me nor did it bother me any. I couldn't help it if I had to blink. Every time I blink is like a chance for my eyes to rest. I just figured my eyes got tired more than most others', and that would make sense, because my eyes strain in order to see. People tell me my blink rate is closer to normal since the stem cell treatments.

Junior year was about to begin. No one at school knew I had gone to China for stem cells; they thought it was just for family purposes. I chose not to tell people at school because I wasn't sure of what to expect and not sure what others would think of me. Little by little I knew they'd find out and questions would be coming like crazy. I didn't mind, I was just hoping I had a good story to tell them. I was hoping by the time school started I would have greater improvements.

It was soon to be my sixteenth birthday. For any girl, her sixteenth birthday is a time to remember. Most girls want a big party, lots of friends and family around, and of course a new car. I could have all of those things, but I was not sure if a car was in the picture. We went to the eye doctor for my yearly checkup, but didn't mention anything about the China trip.

The doctor didn't pay much attention to us and just did the regular tests. He claimed everything was normal and was the same as in previous years. He said there was nothing he could do about it and refused to do further testing. I wanted further testing to be done because I knew I had some sort of improvements. This doctor was rude and in a hurry to get to his next patient. We felt as though we weren't getting the proper care and decided to transfer eye doctors. I could not get an appointment for another few months.

When it came to my sixteenth birthday, I knew a car was not going to be waiting for me when I woke up. I knew at this point I wouldn't be able to drive. It gave me a sinking feeling to know I couldn't be like the others in my class. I couldn't drive like everyone else. I wanted to drive more than anything. Everyone who's known me since elementary school knew that I'd be one of those girls who would have a big party and car for her sixteenth birthday. That was not happening now.

But instead of a car, my parents tried to find a way to make up for it. They knew how much it hurt to know that I couldn't drive. Mt parents wanted to make this day as special as possible. It was going to be a memorable birthday no matter what. I ended up having a dance party at a nice banquet hall with tons of people, a DJ, and everything else I could want. We went all out for the party and had a terrific time!

On my mom's side of the family, I have other cousins who are affected with LHON as well. But none of their parents seem as willing as my own parents to try treatments for a cure. It could have been because they didn't have the money or time, but to me it seemed as though they weren't as motivated. This just makes me so thankful and grateful for the parents I have. I can never thank them enough for everything that they have done for me to try to help me. God has truly blessed me with wonderful parents. I know when the time comes for another treatment; they would be ready to take that risk once again.

My vision stayed pretty much the same with slight improvements here and there. I didn't need to read Braille anymore, which I thought was an improvement in itself. Before, my main way to read materials was through Braille, but now I was able to use large print or standard font. It was exciting to notice the differences and could not help but hope for more. I was able to see the board if I was sitting fairly close and there wasn't a glare. It had to be written with a black marker, but regardless, I was able to read it. It made a difference in my everyday learning. Others might not have noticed it, but I surely did.

I thought I was the only one who noticed these subtle improvements. But I was wrong. Family, friends, and teachers started to notice that I was doing things a little differently. Many had no idea of what was going on, but were happy to know I was able to see certain things. One teacher said, "Michell, I'm glad I can finally read your handwriting now. You're starting to write bigger than before. Why is that?" I didn't even know how to answer. Before, I used to write really small, it was neat, but it was too small. It was so small that I myself couldn't read it. Now that I wasn't relying on assistive technology as much, I was forced to write in a size in which I could read.

Soon enough, it was time for all of those regular checkups again, one of which was an eye doctor's appointment. I did the usual checkup and everything was going well, but this time he noticed that I was able to see the chart slightly better than before. He knew it wouldn't really be correctable with glasses, but thought it was worth giving it a try. So I tried different lenses to see if anything worked. Surprisingly enough, glasses did make a difference in my vision. With correction, I no longer met the legally blind point. Glasses were only used to help me see things far away. They were beneficial to my seeing the board, signs, and anything coming towards me.

I know my vision is far from perfect and I don't know if it ever will. I sometimes wish I had perfect vision again. I wonder what life would be like if I didn't have LHON. Would things be better? Would they be worse? It's hard to say. Now that I think about it, I wouldn't want to change the life I'm living in for the world. I am happy to be who I am. Being visually impaired has definitely been a struggle for me most of my life and I am still struggling day to day. But it has made me who I am. It has made me become a better person.

Before, people viewed me as self-centered and often called me stuck up. They told me that I only cared about myself. I didn't think about people who weren't as good as me because I felt they weren't worthy. I didn't associate myself with those who were different in any way because I knew I was better than them. I judged people by first glance. I talked about others. Looking back, I realized how wrong I truly was. Life was more than just me. Life was full of surprises, both good and bad. God showed me the true meaning of life.

Everything that I thought wouldn't happen to me happened. Most people would say it was bad karma, but I say it was God's path for me all along. I was the one who became different and suddenly people didn't want to associate with me. I was judged before others even met me. I was made fun of and looked down upon. Life was hard at first, but I had to learn to persevere. And after realizing all of my mistakes from the past, I just had to make things different now. I couldn't change the past, but instead I could learn from it.

Now that I'm about to graduate from high school, I learned to have a new perspective on life. I learned not to look down or judge other people if they're different. Something bad had to happen to me in order for me to realize that everyone is different in their own way. No two people are alike. That's what makes us special.

As the only visually-impaired student at Clovis North, I found that many people view me as their inspiration. I have gone through so much in life. Anyone can do anything if they put their mind to it. I've learned to be empathetic towards others and their feelings. I am trustworthy and will always be there for anyone and everyone. People know what I had to go through, and I am willing to tell anyone if they take the time to ask

It is important to become a stronger person through the obstacles life throws your way. I feel it's important to share with others around you the struggles you've gone through, because in this world no one is ever alone. Many people have the same or similar situations, but may be too afraid to tell you. If you are willing to share, you realize what a small world it actually is. That is why I have been willing in most situations to tell people about the obstacles I had to go through to be the person I am today. Whether or not they have had a similar experience, I believe I am an inspiration to a select few, if not more. Even if I'm not, it's important to me for people to get to know who I really am.

***Michell is currently a junior at Fresno Pacific University studying Psychology

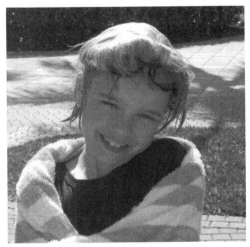
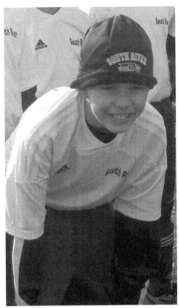

Hope—Our Pioneer

My youngest son Grant was playing quietly in his room one evening. He looked up at me and said, "Mom, my right eye isn't working." Having a blind brother and a visually impaired older son, this was a blow to my soul. In that instant I knew. Leber's Disease was coming for my 8 year old. Dear God, not again. I didn't have the emotional strength to face this.

When he went to bed, I immediately hit the computer again, looking for any information I could find on the "drops" Lissa Poincenot had mentioned at dinner a year earlier. Bingo. I could not find much, but I did find a copy of a letter of request from Dr. Alfredo Sadun to the FDA for permission to use a new drug. It was dated about a year prior.

The next day Grant went for a field test at Dr. Joanne Brilliant's. Sure enough, his right eye had severe central vision loss. His left eye was clear. The only thing I knew was that we had to immediately go see Dr. Sadun. I waited on East Coast time for the office at The University of Southern California to open. When I finally got through, we got an appointment for two weeks later. I also made one for my older son, Chase, since we would be flying there anyway.

Those two weeks were the longest of my life. I walked around in a zombie daze, simply occupying time. Throughout the days I would stop and grab onto something and cry for 10 minutes, then go back to the zombie daze.

Finally, it was time to head to Los Angeles. I had a briefcase full of paperwork: my brother's DNA test, years of Chase's and my brother's field tests, and Grant's singular field test. Finally, I would be meeting a true LHON specialist whom I had idolized for years.

When we arrived, Grant and Chase both went through the battery of neuro-ophthalmologic examinations. The sun shone upon us that day by the pure coincidence that Dr. Valerio Carelli, the world's most foremost pediatric LHON doctor, happened to be visiting the eye center. With the combined team of Dr. Sadun and Dr. Carelli onsite that day, we were under the highest degree of care possible.

Around 1 p.m. a team of about 10 doctors came in to discuss Grant's results. Yes, Leber's Disease had started. The DNA Mutation 14484 was back in action. Grant's field tests had worsened in the last two weeks and visual deficiencies were exhibiting in the left eye also. Dr Sadun stopped at that point and asked if I had any questions. I looked at him and said, "Well, do you want me to go right for the million dollar one?"

"Sure," he replied. I asked was there any possibility of Grant receiving the medication referenced in the paper. He said, "Possibly, we are going to discuss that." My heart soared on even the "maybe." Before then, there had never been anything a patient could do except sit around and learn to be blind. At that time, and up to this day, nothing could be done to help Chase.

We learned there was an orphan drug, but many steps would need to be taken. First, it was necessary Dr.'s Sadun and Carelli agree Grant was a candidate. Next, the drug company would have to approve Grant's acceptance. Finally, the FDA would have to approve him to take it. We would have to stay in Los Angeles a few more days. We had tickets to fly home that evening which we had absolutely no problem ripping to shreds.

While we were celebrating, we also had inherent reservations. We learned Grant would only be the fourth LHON patient if approved. We would be administering an orphan drug, new and untested to Grant. There was no way of predicting if mild or serious unpredictable side effects would occur. While it was difficult to make the decision to place our child on such a medication, the other option was to watch him quickly become blind. There was and still is no option for his brother, or my brother to try this medicine; but, maybe someday.

One problem with testing any potential medications for LHON is that LHON does not have an animal model. Whatever your beliefs may be for animal testing, try grappling with the emotions of giving your child a medication that has not even been tested on a mouse. Your kid is the mouse.

Most readers will have the good fortune of never having read an orphan drug contract; particularly not one containing the words "single patient use under emergency investigation new drug." Nothing drives home the reality and severity of the situation you face like reading "The experimental x drug is being offered because your physicians feel that you have an ophthalmological disease which will cause blindness, and because your physicians have no treatments for this disease." Not that any of this is new information being received, but there is no way to sugarcoat those words or the situation when you are seeing them in a Government document.

The second day of our office visit involved telephone conferences between many parties, filling out paper work, and waiting for the FDA's response. Late in the day Grant received approval and would start the medication the following morning. Once again, the stars had aligned for us. The other three patients had exhibited promising results, but none had started nearly as quickly from the onset of LHON. Grant started the medication 4 weeks from the initial onset of LHON. His initial batch of medication had to be "borrowed" from another patient. Each batch of medicine was produced for the individual patient.`

On this, and on subsequent visits, his 75 pound body had an initial morning blood draw of 3-5 tubes of blood followed by hourly blood draws up until 5 p.m. He gets EKG's every time. He is subjected to the battery of various eye tests. He does it all with the best patient attitude anyone could ever begin to hope for. Grant started the medication on September 9th, 2010. His only complaint was that it tasted disgusting. He had to squirt it in his mouth and eat it with a fatty food 3x a day. His only request was could they possibly give it a new, pleasant flavor.

Our first follow-up visit was scheduled for 4 weeks later. Back at home, in less than a week's time, Grant told us his eyes were getting better. At such an early time-frame, we questioned whether a placebo effect was occurring. With each passing day though, he touted improvement. Home administered tests seemed to be indicating his assessments were accurate. For instance, covering one eye and asking him what various different words across a room were, or what a street sign said.

At the 4-week mark, Grant and I boarded the airplane destined yet again for Los Angeles. The results of his first follow-up visit were remarkable. Grant's recovery was complete and had occurred within 4 weeks. We could hear the excited doctors through the exam room doors. The situation was miraculous. Dr. Sadun quoted to me one of his favorite sayings, "There is no greater thrill than a shot fired, and a bullet dodged." Grant's body had just dodged a bullet. The question that now remained was would it hold.

Grant presented a unique medical research opportunity considering his brother had been affected at a similar age. They are identical mitochondrial twins—each with mutation 14484—so barring the medicine, Grant and Chase should have followed a similar course. There is no comparison in the health of their eyes. One brother is normal, the other visually impaired. Grant was recently part of the published medical article *Effect of EPI-743 on the Clinical Course of the Mitochondrial Disease Leber's Hereditary Optic Neuropathy* by Dr. Alfredo Sadun and eight other doctors. There will eventually be another article comparing my two sons.

Grant has been on the medication for 2 years now. His vision is perfect. While some other patients have been documented to have some recovery, once the disease has started, residual damage can be detected through thorough ophthalmology examinations. There is absolutely no detectable damage to Grant's eyes to this day. Is he the first and only person in the world ever cured? Well, as Dr. Sadun stated to me, "He is a pioneer; therefore, we just don't know, but that is the hope."

Postscript

At this point in time, there is no cure for LHON. It will be many years before this or any other treatment is available to patients. Because of the devastation this disease wreaks on its victims, there are several doctors racing for ways to stop or cure this. If you wish to help our cause, visit the website below and donations can be made online. More information is also available there.

http://www.lhon.org/lhon/LHON.html

Medical Appendix By Dr Edward Chu

Mitochondria and Leber's hereditary optic neuropathy

This chapter aims to provide a basic understanding of the nature, function and importance of mitochondria, relationship between mitochondria and Leber's hereditary optic neuropathy (LHON) as well as the pathology, clinical features and treatment of LHON.

Mitochondria: The Basics

Knowledge of mitochondria is critical to understanding LHON. Mitochondria (or mitochondrion (singular)) is an important organelle (or subunit) found in the cytoplasm, essential in the normal function of a cell. Structurally, a mitochondrion has two layers of lipid membrane, outer and inner membrane. The main purpose of mitochondria is to provide energy and have been called the power plant of cells. If any defect in the mitochondria is present, cells will start to function abnormally due to inadequate energy and this may be a component of mitochondrial diseases. An analogy is a car not functioning due to the absence of gas. Food that we eat is broken down to its simplest form in the stomach and intestines, absorbed into the blood, transported and processed inside each of our cells. From the cytoplasm of the cell, the "processed food" enters the electron transport chain (ETC) of the mitochondria. The ETC is comprised of 5 complexes that, in an assembly line, move electrons off of the food residue (carbon molecule) and onto oxygen. This leads to the production of ATP, for the body to use as energy source. This process is called oxidative phosphorylation. In certain situation, such as intense exercise, or pathology, such as ischemia (lack of blood supply), the body can use an alternative but inefficient pathway that produce less ATP and generates lactic acid as a by-product. In addition to the issue of ATP production, mitochondria can become dysfunctional especially if exposed to constant unfavorable conditions. If damage to cells become irreversible, the mitochondria can initiate a process called apoptosis or programmed cell death.

It is important to understand that mitochondria carry some of their own DNA, called mitochondrial DNA (mtDNA). mtDNA is different to the DNA found in the nucleus of cells. During fertilization (when the egg and sperm unite to form a zygote and eventually a fetus), mitochondria from the egg (from the mother) are passed along and eventually become the mitochondria of the fetus. However, the mitochondria from the sperm are not transferred to the offspring. Hence, mitochondria found in subsequent generations are always maternal in origin and generally speaking, siblings from the same mother are technically identical twins in consideration of the mtDNA.

So how does this relate to LHON? The transmission of the LHON mutation is always maternal in origin (mother to all sons and daughters). To put it in another way, the son will never pass on the mutation to his offspring unless the son marries a woman with a LHON mutation. But the daughter will always pass this genetic condition along.

Leber's hereditary optic neuropathy (LHON)

LHON is one of a number of conditions called mitochondrial diseases. Apart from LHON, other mitochondrial diseases that are very devastating (not limited to this list) include myoneurogenic gastrointestinal encephalopathy, myoclonic epilepsy with ragged red fibers, Leigh disease and mitochondrial encephalomyopathy, lactic acidosis, and stroke-like episodes.

LHON is the most common mitochondrial disease (Man et al, 2003). It affects the optic nerve and retinal ganglion cells that eventually lead to blindness. Around 15 in 100,000 carry the LHON mtDNA mutation (Sadun et al, 2011). In terms of visual loss from LHON, it is estimated to be at 1 in 30,000 in Northeast England while in the Netherlands and Finland, the occurrence is around 1 in 40,000 and 1 in 50,000, respectively (Man et al, 2003; Spruijt et al, 2006; Puomila et al, 2007). Generally, the greatest risk of blindness is commonly seen in males between ages of 15-35 years old (Fraser et al, 2010), however an exception to this is in women who reached menopause (Giordano et al, 2011).

Theodor Leber, a German ophthalmologist, was the first to describe this disease in 1871 (Leber, 1871). To the uninitiated, Leber's hereditary optic neuropathy (LHON) sounds similar to Leber's congenital amaurosis (LCA), which was also described by the same ophthalmologist in 1869 (Leber, 1869). But LCA is totally unrelated and should not be confused with LHON. They affect different tissue in different ways, at different ages and the treatment of one is not effective in the other. It was not until 1988 that Wallace et al discovered that point mutation of the mtDNA was the cause of LHON (Wallace et al, 1988).

There are three common LHON mutations, named after the nucleotide position that harbors the mutation: 3460, 14484 and 11778 and these three mutations comprise almost 95% of LHON patients (Carelli et al, 2004, Fraser et al, 2010, Yu-Wai-Man et al, 2011). Knowledge of the type of mutation is essential as the latter is a factor to determine the prognosis of spontaneous visual improvement, with 14484 having the most favorable outcome. Johns et al reported that recovery from vision loss occurs in 37% of LHON patients with the 14484 mutation (Johns et al, 1993). Other studies reported visual improvements in 14484 patients from 64% to 71% (Spruijt et al, 2006; Mackey et al, 1992; Riordan-Eva et al, 1995). Recovery from vision loss in 11778 occurs in about 4% (Stone et al, 1992) to 22% (Spruijt et al, 2006) while patients with 3460 mutation occurs in 15% (Spruijt et al, 2006) to 20% (Johns et al, 1992). Furthermore, spontaneous visual improvements was observed to occur more than 1 year after vision loss but unusual to occur within 1 year or after 4 years following loss of vision (Spruijt et al, 2006; Johns et al, 1993).

Important terms in LHON and risk factors to becoming blind in LHON

A majority of people with the LHON mutation may not know they have the mutation until they or one of their family members becomes blind. Furthermore, having the mutation is necessary but not sufficient to cause blindness (Sadun et al, 2012). These individuals with the mutation who still see well are called carriers. In those who have the mutation and are blind in either one or both eyes are called affected. Conversion is a term used in LHON whereby a carrier becomes affected. These terms are important and useful in the treatment of LHON. Conversion occurs more in males than females. In a well—studied Brazilian family with 11778, conversion occurs in 45% in males in comparison to 10% in females (Sadun et al, 2003). In addition to gender, conversion can occur when an individual with LHON is exposed to certain factors. These include 1) environmental such as exposure to smoke not limited to cigarettes but also to tire fires, wood camp fires and grills (ie barbeque), malfunctioning stoves as well as excessive consumption of alcohol (Sadun et al, 2002; Sadun et al, 2003; Sanchez et al, 2006); 2) medications, specifically some chronically used antimicrobials such as ethambutol, linezolid, chloramphenicol, streptomycin, zidovudine (including other antiretroviral drugs) and other aminoglycosides (De Marinis, 2001; Ikeda et al, 2006; Sadun et al, 2011); 3) toxins such as pesticides, cyanide and methanol (Sadun et al, 2011); 4) nutritional deficiencies such as deficiencies in vitamin B12, folate and certain amino acids such as cysteine and methionine (Sadun et al, 2012).

Mechanism of LHON

How does the LHON mutation cause the disease? The LHON mutation affects the complex 1 of the ETC and subsequent blocks the shuttling of electrons from complex 1 to complex 3. This leads to decreased oxidative phosphorylation and subsequent decrease in ATP (Carelli et al, 2004; Fraser et al, 2010). Furthermore, cells of LHON have a higher level of reactive oxygen species (ROS). The combined effect of decreased ATP and elevated ROS can damage and eventually lead to RGC and optic nerve death in LHON.

Diagnosis and Clinical features

LHON is usually diagnosed clinically but confirmation can be made with a blood test to detect one of the three common mtDNA mutation (Sadun et al, 2011). However, when the blood test is negative and the symptoms and signs are still suggestive of LHON, the diagnosis of LHON should still be considered, as about 5% of cases are not due to these common mutations (Sadun et al, 2011).

A common scenario in LHON is a male college freshman, with no previous eye problems, who suddenly complains of decrease vision in one eye commonly described as a smudge in their central vision. Further questioning of the patient reveals typical scenarios such as binge drinking or heavy exposure to smoke 6 to 8 weeks earlier. Furthermore, there is often a male family member, related on the maternal side, who became blind at a young age with a vague or unclear diagnosis. On examination, there is a reduction in visual acuity, color perception and brightness sense (Carelli et al, 2004). Fundus examination (looking at the back of the eye) sometimes shows pseudo-edema of the optic disc, circumpapillary telangiectatic *microangiopathy* and swelling of the retinal nerve fiber layer with temporal atrophy of the optic nerve (Carelli et al, 2004; Fraser et al, 2010). However, at times, the fundus can appear normal. Visual field testing usually reveals a central or cecocentral scotoma (Carelli et al, 2004; Sadun et al, 2011). Depending on course of the disease, optical coherence tomography or OCT of the retinal nerve fiber layer reveals swelling in the superior and inferior quadrants, and thinning as the disease progresses (Barboni et al, 2010). Most of the time, this individual will have a tentative diagnosis of optic neuritis and be treated with intravenous steroid with no improvement (Sadun et al, 2012). MRI of the brain and cerebrospinal fluid examination is normal (Sadun et al, 2012). Unfortunately, the other eye will also become involved. This will lead to a referral to a neuro-ophthalmologist and eventually a diagnosis of LHON will be made (Sadun et al, 2012).

Treatment

In the past, a diagnosis of LHON, similar to other mitochondrial diseases, is often devastating as treatment is unavailable. To date, there is still no approved therapy for LHON, however, there are now potential medications that are currently being studied. These agents, idebenone and EPI-743, are under a general class of therapy called quinones (Sadun et al, 2011; Sadun et al, 2012). The use of quinone originated from co-enzyme Q10 (CoQ10), which is not only a nutritional supplement but also a substance found in the ETC that shuttles electron from complex I to complex III. As discussed earlier, the LHON mutation results to defect in complex I that leads to decrease electron transfer and subsequently decrease in ATP production. It was thought that CoQ10 could overcome this impaired shuttling of electrons and for some time CoQ10 was used to treat LHON patients. However, since CoQ10 has a long phospholipid tail and the ETC is surrounded by a lipid membrane, CoQ10 is unable to enter the ETC to assist the shuttling impairment (Geromel et al, 2002). In short, it can't be delivered to where it would be useful.

To overcome this problem, a second-generation quinone, idebenone, with a shorter phospholipid tail was developed (Enns et al, 2012). This allows idebenone to enter the mitochondria and subsequently shuttle electron across the defect. Improvement of vision with idebenone has been reported in a number of cases (Mashima et al, 2000; Sabet-Peyman et al, 2012). More convincingly, two major studies revealed that idebenone has therapeutic benefits (Klopstock et al, 2011; Carelli et al, 2011). The first, a prospective study done by Klopstock and colleagues, included 85 patients with LHON. Fifty-five patients were given 900mg per day while 30 patients were given placebo for 6 months. Visual recovery was minor, but almost achieved statistical significance (Klopstock et al, 2011). The second, a retrospective study done by Carelli and associates involved 103 LHON patients (Carelli et al, 2011). Forty-four patients were treated with idebenone for 1-5 years and noted mild visual recovery mainly in 11778 patients that was statistically significant (Carelli et al, 2011). Unfortunately to inadequate data, it was not possible to determine the response of the other two LHON mutations (3460 and 14484) to idebenone.

Another medication that is currently being studied is a third generation quinone called EPI-743. Like other quinones, it shuttles electrons from complex I to complex III and is also a strong antioxidant (Shrader et al, 2011; Enns et al, 2012; Sadun et al, 2012—EPI-743). The latter is likely beneficial in LHON as these cells have higher than normal reactive oxygen species (ROS) that are detrimental. Antioxidants may neutralize these harmful ROS preventing cell death. It was noted in cell cultures that EPI-743 is more effective than idebenone (Sadun et al, 2012—EPI-743). Recently, Sadun and coworkers published a paper on 5 LHON patients taking EPI-743 (Sadun et al, 2012—EPI-743). Four out of the 5 patients revealed improvement in visual acuity, visual fields and retinal nerve fiber layer via OCT. Furthermore, normalization of vision was seen in two of these patients.

The use of combination therapy may not be advantageous for quinones and might actually be detrimental. Quinones can bind and compete for the same site. If one takes idebenone or EPI-743 with CoQ10, there is a possibility that some of the idebenone or EPI-743 will be displaced by CoQ10 and not be absorbed by the body.

Menopausal women, who are carriers of LHON, may benefit from estrogen (hormone replacement therapy) (Giordano et al, 2011). Such a decision must be coordinated with a gynecologist or primary care physician as there are complicated risks as well as benefits in taking such hormonal replacement therapy.

References:

Man PY, Griffiths PG, Brown DT, Howell N, Turnbull DM, Chinnery PF. The epidemiology of Leber hereditary optic neuropathy in the North East of England. Am J Hum Genet. 2003;72:333-339.

Sadun AA, La Morgia C, Carelli V. Leber's Hereditary Optic Neuropathy. Curr Treat Options Neurol. 2011;13:109-117.

Spruijt L, Kolbach DN, de Coo RF, Plomp AS, Bauer NJ, Smeets HJ, de Die-Smulders CE. Influence of mutation type on clinical expression of Leber hereditary optic neuropathy. Am J Ophthalmol. 2006;141:676-682.

Puomila A, Hämäläinen P, Kivioja S, Savontaus ML, Koivumäki S, Huoponen K, Nikoskelainen E. Epidemiology and penetrance of Leber hereditary optic neuropathy in Finland. Eur J Hum Genet. 2007;15:1079-1089.

Fraser JA, Biousse V, Newman NJ. The neuro-ophthalmology of mitochondrial disease. Surv Ophthalmol. 2010;55:299-334.

Giordano C, Montopoli M, Perli E, Orlandi M, Fantin M, Ross-Cisneros FN, Caparrotta L, Martinuzzi A, Ragazzi E, Ghelli A, Sadun AA, d'Amati G, Carelli V. Oestrogens ameliorate mitochondrial dysfunction in Leber's hereditary optic neuropathy. Brain. 2011;134:220-234.

Leber Th. Ueber hereditaere und congenital angelegte sehnervenleiden. Graefes Arch Ophthalmol. 1871;17:249-291.

Leber Th. Ueber Retinitis pigmentosa und angeborene Amaurose. Graefes Arch Ophthalmol. 1869;15:1-25.

Wallace DC, Singh G, Lott MT, Hodge JA, Schurr TG, Lezza AM, Elsas LJ 2nd, Nikoskelainen EK. Mitochondrial DNA mutation associated with Leber's hereditary optic neuropathy. Science. 1988;242:1427-30.

Carelli V, Ross-Cisneros FN, Sadun AA: Mitochondrial dysfunction as a cause of optic neuropathies. Prog Retin Eye Res. 2004;23:53-89.

Yu-Wai-Man P, Griffiths PG, Chinnery PF. Mitochondrial optic neuropathies —disease mechanisms and therapeutic strategies. Prog Retin Eye Res. 2011;30:81-114.

Johns DR, Heher KL, Miller NR, Smith KH. Leber's hereditary optic neuropathy. Clinical manifestations of the 14484 mutation. Arch Ophthalmol. 1993;111:495-498.

Mackey D, Howell N. A variant of Leber hereditary optic neuropathy characterized by recovery of vision and by an unusual mitochondrial genetic etiology. Am J Hum Genet. 1992;51:1218-1228.

Riordan—Eva P, Sanders MD, Govan GG, Sweeney MC, DaCosta J, Harding AE. The clinical features of Leber's hereditary optic neuropathy defined by the presence of a pathogenic mitochondrial DNA mutation. Brain. 1995;118:319-337.

Stone EM, Newman NJ, Miller NR, Johns DR, Lott MT, Wallace DC. Visual recovery in patients with Leber's hereditary optic neuropathy and the 11778 mutation. J Clin Neuro-ophthalmol 1992;12:10-14.

Johns DR, Smith KH, Miller NR. Leber's hereditary optic neuropathy. Clinical manifestations of the 3460 mutation.Arch Ophthalmol. 1992;110:1577-1581.

Sadun AA, La Morgia C, Carelli V. Leber's hereditary optic neuropathy: new quinone therapies change the paradigm. Expert Rev Ophthalmol. 2012;7:251-259.

Sadun AA, Carelli V, Salomao SR, et al.: Extensive investigation of a large Brazilian pedigree of 11778/haplogroup J Leber hereditary optic neuropathy. Am J Ophthalmol. 2003;136:231-238.

Sadun AA, Carelli V, Salomao SR, et al.: A very large Brazilian pedigree with 11778 Leber's hereditary optic neuropathy. Trans Am Ophthalmol Soc. 2002;100:169-178. discussion 178-179.

Sanchez RN, Smith AJ, Carelli V, Sadun AA, Keltner JL. Leber hereditary optic neuropathy possibly triggered by exposure to tire fire. J Neuroophthalmol. 2006;26:268-272.

De Marinis M. Optic neuropathy after treatment with anti-tuberculous drugs in a subject with Leber's hereditary optic neuropathy mutation. J Neurol. 2001;248:818-819.

Ikeda A, Ikeda T, Ikeda N, et al.: Leber's hereditary optic neuropathy precipitated by ethambutol. Jpn J Ophthalmol. 2006;50:280-283.

Barboni P, Carbonelli M, Savini G, et al.: Natural history of Leber's hereditary optic neuropathy: longitudinal analysis of the retinal nerve fiber layer by optical coherence tomography. Ophthalmology. 2010;117:623-627.

Geromel V, Darin N, Chrétien D, Bénit P, DeLonlay P, Rötig A, Munnich A, Rustin P. Coenzyme Q(10) and idebenone in the therapy of respiratory chain diseases: rationale and comparative benefits. Mol Genet Metab. 2002;77:21-30.

Enns GM, Kinsman SL, Perlman SL, Spicer KM, Abdenur JE, Cohen BH, Amagata A, Barnes A, Kheifets V, Shrader WD, Thoolen M, Blankenberg F, Miller G. Initial experience in the treatment of inherited mitochondrial disease with EPI-743. Mol Genet Metab. 2012;105:91-102.

Mashima Y, Kigasawa K, Wakakura M, Oguchi Y. Do idebenone and vitamin therapy shorten the time to achieve visual recovery in Leber hereditary optic neuropathy? J Neuroophthalmol. 2000;20:166-170.

Sabet-Peyman EJ, Khaderi KR, Sadun AA. Is Leber hereditary optic neuropathy treatable? Encouraging results with idebenone in both prospective and retrospective trials and an illustrative case. J Neuroophthalmol. 2012;32:54-57.

Klopstock T, Yu-Wai-Man P, Dimitriadis K, Rouleau J, Heck S, Bailie M, Atawan A, Chattopadhyay S, Schubert M, Garip A, Kernt M, Petraki D, Rummey C, Leinonen M, Metz G, Griffiths PG, Meier T, Chinnery PF. A randomized placebo-controlled trial of idebenone in Leber's hereditary optic neuropathy. Brain. 2011;134:2677-2686.

Carelli V, La Morgia C, Valentino ML, Rizzo G, Carbonelli M, De Negri AM, Sadun F, Carta A, Guerriero S, Simonelli F, Sadun AA, Aggarwal D, Liguori R, Avoni P, Baruzzi A, Zeviani M, Montagna P, Barboni P. Idebenone treatment in Leber's hereditary optic neuropathy. Brain. 2011;134:e1-5.

Shrader WD, Amagata A, Barnes A, Enns GM, Hinman A, Jankowski O, Kheifets V, Komatsuzaki R, Lee E, Mollard P, Murase K, Sadun AA, Thoolen M, Wesson K, Miller G. α-Tocotrienol quinone modulates oxidative stress response and the biochemistry of aging. Bioorg Med Chem Lett. 2011;21:3693-3698.

Sadun AA, Chicani CF, Ross-Cisneros FN, Barboni P, Thoolen M, Shrader WD, Kubis K, Carelli V, Miller G. Effect of EPI-743 on the clinical course of the mitochondrial disease Leber hereditary optic neuropathy. Arch Neurol. 2012;69:331-338.

About the Author

Valerie Rudisill lives in Annapolis, Md. She discovered she suffered from an extremely rare Mitochondrial Disease in 1999. The disease causes permanent blindness. Many family members have since suffered. Currently she is a carrier, but that can change at any moment. A life changing event in October 2010 inspired this book. The book would not be possible without the help of effected others who kindly shared their stories. She hopes this book will aide and inspire people. One day she hopes a cure will exist for all suffering from this disease.

9033936R00142

Made in the USA
San Bernardino, CA
02 March 2014